Homoeopathic Remedies for Middle and Old Age

Health Care in
Orient Paperbacks

The Complete Book of Family Homoeopathic Medicine *(Illus.)*
The Complete Book of Home Remedies *(Illus.)*
Magnetic Cure for Common Diseases *(Illus.)*
Yogic Cure for Common Diseases *(Illus.)*
Nature Cure for Common Diseases
Accupressure Cure for Common Diseases *(Illus.)*
Home Guide to Medical Emergencies *(Illus.)*
The Complete Family Medicine Book
Mental Tension and Its cure
A-Z of Childhood Illnesses *(Illus.)*
Aromatherapy *(Illus.)*
Herbal Remedies & Home Comforts
A Guide to Herbal Remedies
Healing with Gems & Crystals
Asthma Self-Help Book

Homoeopathic Remedies
FOR MIDDLE & OLD AGE

Dr Keith M. Souter
MB, ChB, MRCGP, MHMA

Index compiled by Lyn Greenwood

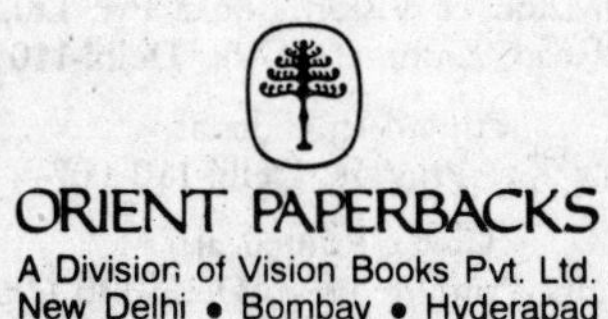

ORIENT PAPERBACKS
A Division of Vision Books Pvt. Ltd.
New Delhi • Bombay • Hyderabad

Authorised Edition for sale in
India, Pakistan, Bangladesh & Nepal only

ISBN 81-222-0177-6

1st Published in Orient Paperbacks 1995
2nd Printing 1997

Homoeopathic Remedies for Middle and Old Age

Published in England as
Homoeopathy for the Third Age

Published in arrangement with
The C.W. Daniel Company Ltd., England

Cover Design by Vision Studio

Published by
Orient Paperbacks
(A Division of Vision Books Pvt. Ltd.)
Madarsa Road, Kashmere Gate, Delhi-110 006

Printed in India at
Kay Kay Printers, Delhi-110 007

Cover Printed at
Ravindra Printing Press, Delhi-110 006

Contents

PART THREE: Selecting Appropriate Remedies

The Third Age

The term, The Third Age, has been used in this book to broadly describe what is commonly known as Middle Age and Old Age. The reasons for the author's choice of this term are further elaborated in chapter one.

Introduction

The Third Age should be a time to look forward to. It is the part of one's life when there should be enough time to ease back and enjoy oneself. Unfortunately, however, it is also a time when health problems, bereavements and all sorts of other events crowd in to affect one's sense of well-being.

Orthodox medicine can work wonders in maintaining failing organs and systems. On the other hand, many drugs produce unacceptable side effects, resulting in up to ten per cent of hospital admissions for the over 65s.

Over the last few years more and more people have been turning to homoeopathy as a gentler approach to their health problems. Indeed, for many people in the Third Age it is an ideal method of treatment since it does not throw any strain upon already straining organs and systems, and it is free from harmful side effects.

This book is not intended to replace orthodox medical treatment or advice. Where it is essential to seek medical advice then this is mentioned throughout the text. With many conditions it is as well to inform your medical adviser of any homoeopathic treatment being taken, although there will be no interaction with conventional drugs. Above all, it is important not to stop taking any prescribed medication without consulting your adviser.

There are three parts to the book. Part One covers

general aspects of ageing and the principles of homoeopathy. Part Two deals with problems which are extremely common in the Third Age. Finally, Part Three contains a Materia Medica, an outline of all of the profiles of the remedies used in the book. In addition, there is a Therapeutic Index, an A–Z of common conditions and symptoms detailing the remedies which work well for them.

To get the best out of this book it is as well to read through Part One to understand the basic principles of the method, then turn to Part Two for information about specific problems. The Materia Medica gives a fuller description of the remedies and can be used to check them prior to use. Finally, as a quick reference tool, the Therapeutic Index can guide you to remedies which are probably of use in set conditions. Again, the Materia Medica allows the final check to be made.

There has for many years been a need for a homoeopathic book aimed at people in the Third Age. I hope that this small text will fill that niche and prove useful to individuals, carers and all people involved in helping people in the Third Age.

Keith Souter

PART ONE

Homoeopathy
The Gentle Medicine

1

The Ageing Process

'Which is the animal that has four feet in the morning, two at midday and three in the evening?'

The riddle of The Sphinx

According to mythology the road to Ancient Thebes was guarded by the Sphinx, a fabulous monster with the face and bust of a woman, the body of a lion and the wings of a bird. Travellers who failed to answer her riddle were rapidly devoured. Only Oedipus was able to rise to the challenge.

He answered: 'Man, who in infancy crawls on all fours, who walks on two feet in maturity, and in his old age supports himself with a stick.'

Thus we see that even in antiquity it was accepted that there were three ages of man. The period of infancy as such extended until one was independent enough to 'walk on one's own two feet.' Maturity then lasted while one was useful to society, until the Third Age was heralded by the increasing need to use a crutch of one form or another.

To the Ancient Chinese three ages were not considered enough. In *The Yellow Emperor's Classic of Internal Medicine*, reputedly written over four thousand years ago, seven ages are described for both men and women. Not only that, but whereas the three ages referred to by Oedipus are quite non-specific in terms of time, the Chinese ages were based on cycles of seven years for women and eight years for men.

Shakespeare also considered things to be more complicated than mere growth, maturity and decline. In one of his most famous speeches from the play *As You Like It*, he has Jaques, a lord attending the banished Duke say:

All the world's a stage,
And all the men and women merely players:
They have their exits and their entrances;
And one man in his time plays many parts,
His acts being seven ages.

Jaques then describes the ages of the typical Elizabethan man from 'mewling' infant to middle-aged round-bellied pillar of respectability, full of accumulated wisdom and experience of the world. Then finally as the seventh age dawns:

Last scene of all,
That ends this strange eventful history,
Is second childishness and mere oblivion,
Sans teeth, sans eyes, sans taste, sans everything.

Of course, when we look at categorisations of anything to do with human beings it is obvious that we are imposing quite arbitrary parameters. The Ancient Chinese, for example, deliberately imposed cycles of seven and eight years because these had special significance in the number theory which was an integral part of their philosophy and system of medicine. Similarly, Shakespeare's use of seven ages was really nothing more than a literary device.

But Shakespeare's image of the final phase of life with a reversion to childhood and with increasing failure of all the senses and bodily functions is gloomy beyond mention. Indeed, while it probably was the norm for anyone fortunate enough to survive past 50 years during the Elizabethan era, such should not be the case as we approach the 21st century. Indeed, there is much that the individual can do to maintain optimum health.

Ageing

The ageing process begins at conception and continues until death. This at any rate is what is meant by *biological ageing*, since it potentially includes all the changes that come about through growth and development from fertilised egg to newborn baby, allowing also for maturation to adulthood, and for the secondary effects of illness, disease and natural degeneration.

Generally speaking, however, by 'ageing' we refer to the period of time after the individual has passed his or her biological peak. Further changes are then considered to be deteriorative. Effectively, this is the *Third Age* of man.

Among gerontologists (the scientists who study the ageing process, as opposed to geriatricians who are physicians for the elderly) there is debate about the relevance of biological and chronological age. The two may mean the same thing if an individual seems (biologically) to be as old as his years (chronological age) would suggest. On the other hand some people seem to be older or younger than their years. It would be nice if the correlates were strong enough to predict the life expectancy of the individual on this basis, but this is not the case.

Lifespan and life expectancy

It is a fact that the population structure of Britain and most other developed countries has changed dramatically over the last hundred or so years. Whereas at the turn of this century the proportion of people over the age of 65 was around five per cent, it is now almost seventeen per cent. Admittedly, one has to consider that over this period of time the birth rate has halved, and the number of young people who have died from infectious diseases has dropped considerably. Nevertheless, there are currently more people over the age of 65 than have ever been over 65 since cumulative human history began.

At the time of the Ancient Egyptians 40 years would

have been considered a good age, while 65 would have seemed positively ancient. The Bible tells us that the allotted span was some three score years and ten, although relatively few people would have lived that long. Again, forty years would have been nearer the mark.

There is a distinction to be made here between lifespan and life expectancy. The 'lifespan' is the potential which an individual could live if they are fortunate to be unhampered by accident or disease. As mentioned above, according to the Bible it was 70 years.

'Life expectancy' on the other hand, is a statistical expression of how many years a member of a group with similar life characteristics can expect to live. Using life tables it is then possible to say what the expectation of life is for a certain group at birth or at any specific age. As an example, the life expectation for a female born in Britain in 1841 was 42 years, but if she lived to 65 years her further expectation was 11.6 years. Now, in 1992, the life expectation for a female would be 75 years at birth, and 16 years at 65.

It is further interesting to note that the expectation at 65 did not increase until about 1930. The significance of this is that the number of people living past the age of 75 is getting greater, so that by 2001 it is estimated that there will have been an increase of forty per cent based on figures for 1980. Further, there will have been an increase of fifty per cent for the over 85s.

Current theories about ageing

The fact that everyone ages is obvious. The actual mechanisms whereby this process comes about are still, however, unclear to science. In general, current theories can be classified into three categories:

SYSTEM-DEGENERATION THEORIES

These theories postulate that increasing failure of the immune system, the nervous system or the endocrine (hormonal) system result in loss of the governing function that all of these systems exert over the body.

BIOCHEMICAL THEORIES

These postulate that particular biochemical reactions start to take place which affect certain cells of the body or their function. Worthy of note is the '*Free Radical Theory*.'

Free radicals are molecules with an unpaired electron. During all sorts of normal metabolic processes they occur momentarily. Their significance is that they can produce free radical reactions which are capable of damaging all sorts of biological material, including DNA, proteins, fats and enzymes. Because of this they can disrupt cell membranes and subcellular organelles. It is thought that such free radical reactions become commoner with age. Interestingly, there seems to be some protection offered against them by substances called antioxidants which are present in many types of fruit and green vegetables. Accordingly, we shall return to this subject in chapter five.

DNA-BASED THEORIES

Some of these theories are almost fatalistic, in that they postulate that 'all is written' in the genetic code of the Deoxyribosenucleic acid (DNA) molecule. In other words, the lifespan of the individual is pre-programmed in the nucleic structure of every cell of the body.

Other DNA theories suggest that damage occurs to the DNA molecules with age, so that the controlling effect upon the whole body is somehow affected.

Currently, the orthodox scientific view is that the natural lifespan is set genetically at around 85 years, with a scatter effect so that some individuals may reach 100 and other less than 70.

Ageing changes

All sorts of things are often attributed to 'just getting old.' Similarly, it is often said that it is 'normal to get (such and such) when you're old.' But what exactly does that mean? Is there such a thing as 'normal ageing?'

Medically speaking, normal ageing means growing old in the absence of disease or malformation of any sort. This is really a physiological ideal, wherein the only changes taking place with age are those of slowly diminishing function of different systems.

Some of the more important changes are as follows:

THE CARDIOVASCULAR SYSTEM

The muscle tissue of the heart undergoes some loss and becomes thickened and fibrosed. The effect of this is to cause a reduction in cardiac output (effectively the pumping ability of the heart) by up to 30 per cent of the young adult level by the age of 75.

The heart valves also have a tendency to become hardened with calcium deposition, thereby causing them either to leak or impede the flow of blood.

The electrical conducting tissue of the heart often becomes fibrosed, so that the natural pacemaker of the heart, the *sino-atrial node*, fails to act effectively. The result of this is to produce an irregular beating of the heart with reduced pump effectiveness. The most common variant of this is *atrial fibrillation*, which occurs in about 12 per cent of people over 70.

Finally, hardening of the arteries is usually well advanced by the 50s, often resulting in hypertension, or high blood pressure.

THE BRAIN

The cells of the brain have to last for life, in that they cannot be replaced by new cells as can other tissues of the body. The loss of these cells in fact starts gradually from about the age of 25 years, the rate of loss increasing dramatically after the age of 80.

THE KIDNEYS

The flow of blood to the kidneys falls by 50 per cent by the age of 85 years, as does the filtering ability of the kidney. This is extremely important in the way the body handles, or fails to handle conventional drugs.

THE BOWEL

The blood and nerve supply to the bowel both diminish with age. As a result the absorptive ability of the bowel may become impaired, again resulting in difficulty with the handling of drugs, as well as that of certain vitamins and minerals.

Ageing and disease

As stated earlier, it is difficult to say what is normal ageing and what is due to age-related disease. The fact is that all diseases are commoner the older one becomes. Not only that, but there is a tendency for those in the Third Age to suffer from 'multiple pathology', or from several conditions at once. This pattern plus the coexistent normal ageing changes may tend to alter the expected symptom patterns from any one disease.

Ageing and the mind

It is quite incorrect in my opinion to suggest that there are any 'normal' ageing changes. There may be a tendency for personality traits to become more entrenched, so that the meticulous individual becomes even more meticulous, or the independent-minded become even more so for as long as they can. Confusion, intellectual impairment and dementia, on the other hand, are more likely to be secondary results of affections of the brain.

Situational changes in the individual's life may well be of more importance. Enforced retirement, reduced income, bereavement, isolation, physical illness and loss of independence, all of these can be hard to come to terms with. They can all induce negative states of mind which may contribute to a dropping of resistance and the development of secondary problems, both physical and mental.

Drug Treatment

As mentioned earlier, ageing is associated with a reduction in the physiological functioning of various systems of the body. The kidneys are less efficient filters, the liver metabolises less well, and the bowel's absorptive ability can become quite variable. In addition, the muscle mass of the body is reduced, producing a relative increase in the fat mass. All of these have a potential effect upon the way the body absorbs, reacts to and excretes conventional drugs.

Iatrogenic disease, or man-made disease is common in the Third Age and is usually due to side effects from conventional drug treatment. The more drugs that are taken the more likely is this to be a problem. Indeed, about 10 per cent of all hospital admissions for people in the Third Age are because of such iatrogenic illness.

Age and life

So far we have considered ageing from the biological view. We have seen how different theories attempt to explain the nature of ageing. We have seen that the ageing process is accompanied by an increased incidence of all diseases, and we have seen why we have to be wary of over-using drugs, because of the altered way we handle them as we get older.

The thing is, however, that the theories about ageing (limited as they are) are all very well—provided one accepts the premise that the body is merely a biological machine. They do not explain anything about life itself or the Vital Force which energises us. This above all is the most limiting thing about modern Medicine.

In Homoeopathy the Vital Force is accepted as an integral part of each and every person. Indeed, as science advances it becomes clearer that the emphasis of medicine in the future will have to veer away from the biochemical towards the biophysical. And when this happens homoeopathy will take its place at the forefront of the New Medicine.

2

The Vital Force

Without the vital force the material body is unable to feel, or act, or maintain itself.

Dr Samuel Hahnemann

Orthodox medicine is firmly based upon a biomedical model which views the human body as an intricate machine made up of vast numbers of cells, each of which functions like a tiny biochemical factory. These cells are organised into tissues, the tissues into organs, and the organs into systems. Governing all of this activity is the brain, a biological computer of incredible complexity.

There is much that this model fails to explain. Life in all its myriad forms and complexities is obviously more than mere chemical reactions in cells, spurts of hormones into the blood stream and bursts of electrical nervous activity. Without even considering a spiritual dimension it is surely clear that mere chemistry cannot explain awareness, thought and the whole panoply of emotions which are part and parcel of life.

As we go up the evolutionary ladder from the simplest unicellular organisms, the function of the cells which make up the organism become more specialised and less independent. With fairly complicated organisms whole groups of cells become 'tissues,' sharing a common function which other tissues cannot perform. The extreme form of this is to be found in human nerve cells which are incapable of functioning as anything other than nerve cells because their role is so specialised.

The organisation of cells is something which the

biomedical model fails to explain. Just how do cells develop into one type or another? And once they have developed into a tissue-type what makes them continue to function in a coordinated manner with their neighbours? How do the tissues manage to maintain their integrity?

It is a fact that the cells of the body are constantly dying off and being replaced. Obviously there must be a fine balance between the two, otherwise our tissues and organs would soon degenerate into complete chaos. Is it possible that the neighbouring cells have some sort of 'awareness' of the state of health of a dying cell, perhaps from the release of chemicals, or what? Some sort of control is clearly being exerted, yet the biomedical model fails to adequately explain it.

There is now a growing body of evidence which suggests that the controlling influence is not biochemical but biophysical. It is a form of *Vital Force.*

Vital Force

The concept of some form of Vital Force has been accepted for many centuries by several civilised cultures. The Chinese know it as *Chi* and the Indian yogis as *Prana*. In addition, it has also been postulated or 'rediscovered' by various individuals throughout history. For example, Paracelsus called it *Munia*, the alchemists termed it *Vital Fluid* and Baron Von Reichenbach, the German chemist who discovered creosote, called it *Odyle*. In this century Wilhelm Reich called it *Orgone*.

In all of these cases, although there is a slightly different interpretation, it is regarded as a form of energy which permeates living creatures during life and which is an integral part of their whole being. It is thought to form a field within and around the organism to produce a sort of *etheric body*.

In recent years biophysicists have investigated this etheric body and concluded that it is an energy field, like a plasma constellation of ionised particles. Accordingly, it has been called *biological plasma* or *bioplasma*.

Such an energy system is believed to function as an information system which functions as a template for foetal development, subsequent growth and development, tissue organisation and for trouble-shooting tissue repair. It is effectively an energy double of the physical body which is intricately connected through it as a pervasive, interweaving bioelectronic network, with all the subcellular structures, and organic molecules forming a semi-conductor system.

The subtle anatomy

To say that the etheric body is a double of the physical body is an over-simplification. The two are connected, each one having the potential to affect the other. In terms of health the implication is that illness can arise from direct effects on either the physical or the etheric body.

As mentioned earlier, different medical systems have for centuries been based upon the concept of a Vital Force. From my work in acupuncture and yoga I believe that the models used by these systems provide valuable insights into *the subtle anatomy of the etheric body*. While there are undoubted differences between them, because they have been built up from different viewpoints and with different aims in mind, together they help to conceptualise how the Vital Force works to integrate the etheric and physical bodies.

THE ACUPUNCTURE MERIDIAN SYSTEM

According to acupuncture theory Vital Force flows cyclically through the organ systems of the body, along set energy paths called *meridians*, each of which is associated with a different organ. There are fourteen major meridians running through the body, to produce a highly complicated energy network. (Figure 1)

'Blockage' or disruption of the energy flow eventually

produces an imbalance in function, mirrored by malfunction of a particular organ or organ system.

Upon each meridian there are a number of *acupoints*, stimulation of which can tonify, stimulate or harmonise the appropriate organ system by virtue of the effect upon the flow of Vital Force.

THE YOGIC CHAKRA SYSTEM

In Sanskrit, *chakra* means wheel. The chakras are seen as energy wheels or vortices of energy, each one of which is associated with an endocrine organ and is responsible for helping to energise different parts of the physical body. There are seven major chakras situated in a vertical line between the spine and the front of the body, from the coccyx up to the crown. (Figure 2) In addition, there are many minor chakras and multiple *nadis*, fine vibrational filaments of energy flow similar to the meridians of acupuncture.

★ ★ ★

There are undoubtedly cross-over points between these two systems, as indeed there are likely to be even more systems of Vital Force flow throughout the etheric and physical bodies. Research from centres all over the world has already demonstrated the existence of these networks of energy. The time is ripe to consolidate this research and move the emphasis in medicine away from the biochemical towards the biophysical.

The etheric body and illness

If one accepts that the etheric body has organisational and controlling abilities, then it is likely that aberrations in the etheric body, and therefore in the Vital Force, could result in disorganised function in the physical body. So what sort of things could affect the etheric body?

Since the etheric body, or bioplasma, is essentially an

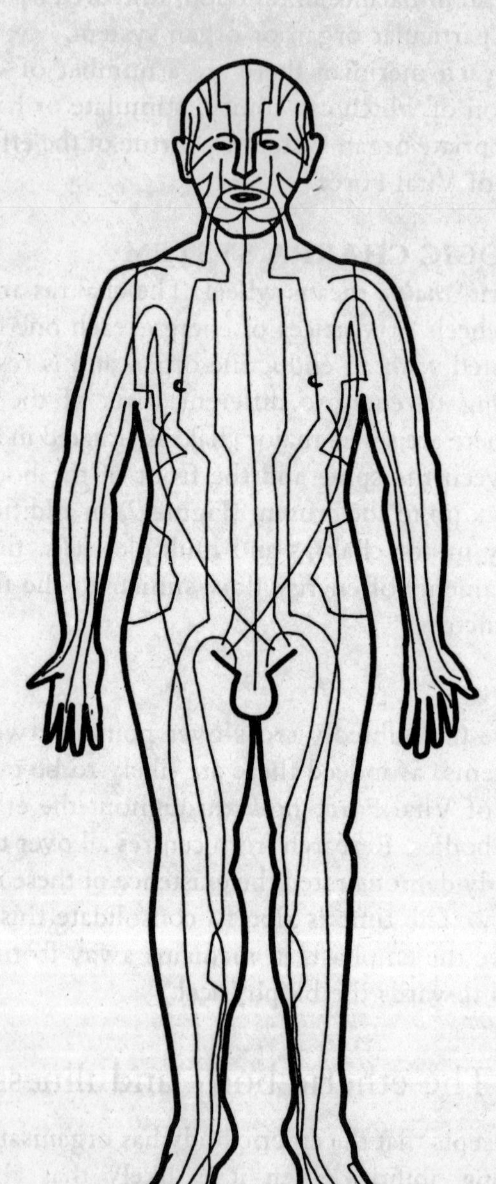

Figure 1. The Meridians of Acupuncture

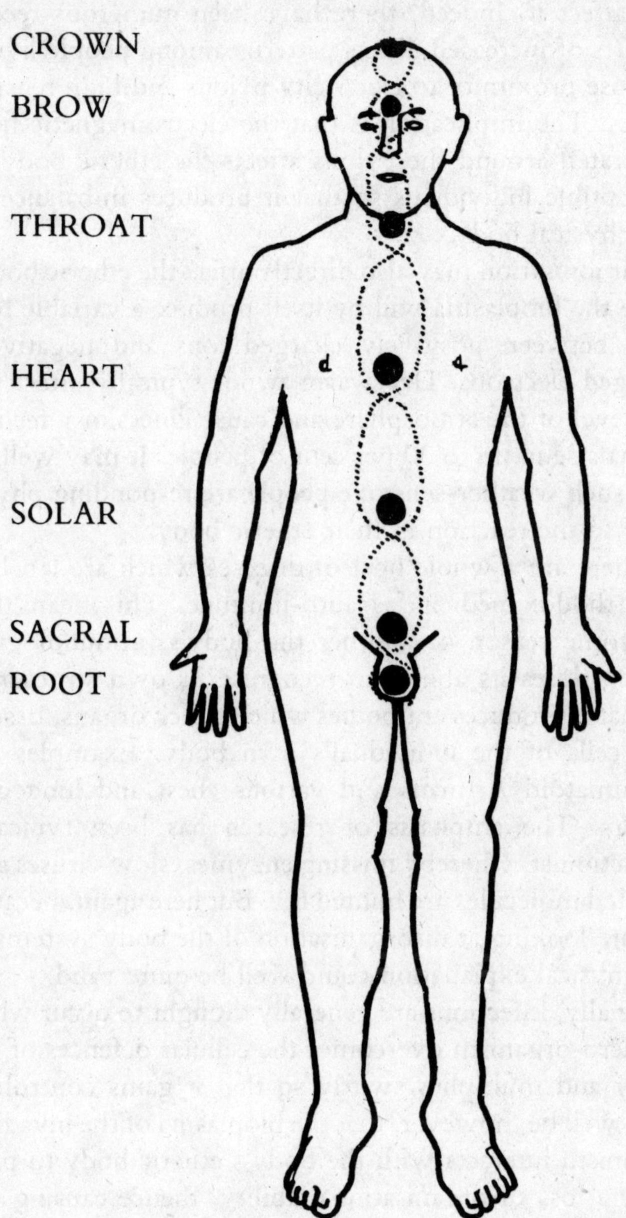

Figure 2. The Chakras

energy field it is quite possible that other energy fields can affect it. Indeed, there have been numerous recent reports of increased illness patterns among people living in close proximity to electricity pylons and high tension cables. The implication is that the electromagnetic field generated around the pylons affects the etheric body of susceptible individuals so that it produces imbalance in the physical body.

Air ionisation may also directly affect the etheric body, since the bioplasma will by itself produce a variable balance between positively charged ions and negatively charged electrons. Dry warm winds typically affect the ion level of the atmosphere and cause illness or a feeling of malaise in up to 30 per cent of people. It may well be that such weather-sensitive people are responding physically to the reaction in their etheric body.

There are a whole host of diseases which are labelled by orthodox medicine as 'auto-immune.' This means that for some reason or another the body's immunological system loses its ability to recognise its own structures, so that it produces antibodies which attack organs, tissues and cells of the individual's own body. Examples are Rheumatoid Arthritis and various chest and lung disorders. The emphasis of research has been typically reductionist, whereby missing enzymes, slow viruses and twisted molecules are hunted for. But here again, because we are looking at disorganisation of the body systems, a biophysical explanation could well be quite valid.

Finally, infections are generally thought to occur when a micro-organism overcomes the cellular defences of the body and multiplies swiftly so that it gains control. It may well be, however, that the bioplasma of the invading organism interacts with the body's etheric body to produce a loss of organisational ability, thence causing the lowered resistance which permits the invader to thrive.

Admittedly, all of these examples are open to debate. The concept I am proposing is that there are circumstances when the causation of illness may lie within the etheric rather than the physical body. When that happens the organisational ability of the etheric body becomes impaired. This impairment then results in the biochemical aberrations which orthodox medicine picks up as 'isolated features.' Essentially, Vital Force and the etheric body fill in many of the gaps created in our understanding when considering the biomedical model alone. They do not replace orthodox theories, but they extend and strengthen them.

The healing power of nature

Hippocrates wrote that physicians did not do anything to heal, but that they helped create the right conditions which would allow nature to heal. He called this innate ability of the body *Vis Medicatrix Naturae* – the healing power of nature.

Few people would doubt this. The surgeon may remove the diseased section of bowel, yet it is for the body to heal the wounds. Similarly, the broken bones may be set, but it is the body that makes them knit together.

People may then say that there are many instances when drugs are necessary to maintain life. Well this is absolutely the case. For instance the insulin-dependent patient must receive his regular insulin, and the patient with chronic heart failure must have his regular medication. These are instances where healing or cure cannot take place and so the aim is maintenance of health. And again that is up to the body.

Yet all of these examples relate to treatment of the physical body. From what has been said before, however, it should be apparent that it may well be possible to treat the individual via the etheric body, by directly stimulating the Vital Force. And indeed, as we shall see in the next chapter it is my belief that this is at the very heart of homoeopathy.

3

How Homoeopathy Works

Similia similibus curentur
(let like be treated by like)

Homoeopathy is a gentle form of medicine which was known to the Ancient Greeks, a fact mirrored by its derivation from the Greek *homoios*, meaning 'like,' and *pathos*, meaning 'suffering.' Essentially it means treating like with like.

It was the great Hippocrates who first taught that there were two ways of treating a patient: either one could cure by 'contraries,' or by 'similarities.' That is, one could either give medication to counteract symptoms—*the law of contraries*; or medication which had the ability to produce the same symptoms as those suffered by the ill person—*the law of similars*.

In both cases he believed that the physician was merely creating the right conditions for the inner healing power, *Vis Medicatrix Naturae* to bring about a cure.

Several hundred years later in sixteenth century Europe, Theophrastus Bombastus von Hohenheim, otherwise known as Paracelsus, threw off the shackles of medical dogmatism and again taught the merits of treating like with like. It was not, however, until the eighteenth century that the basic principles became formalised into a true system of medicine.

Dr Samuel Hahnemann

The founder of this system of medicine was an eccentric genius by the name of Samuel Christian Hahnemann (1755–1843), the son of a china-painter in the famous Meissen pottery works. After qualifying in Medicine from the University of Erlangen in 1779, he practised for several years before becoming disenchanted with the rather brutal and dubious medical treatments of the day. As a result he gave up medical practice, started studying chemistry and eked out a modest living by writing and translating.

In 1790, while translating a textbook written by the eminent Scottish physician Cullen, he came across a section dealing with the treatment of malaria with quinine. Although this was (and still is) an appropriate treatment for the disease, he was unconvinced by Cullen's explanation that it worked by virtue of having a tonic effect upon the stomach. He reasoned that since other more powerful 'tonics' had no such beneficial effect, it had to be working by some other mechanism. Accordingly, experimenter that he was, he dosed himself with quinine for several days, the result being that he began to experience the symptoms of malaria.

Thus the germ of an idea began to form—that a drug which produced the symptoms of an illness in a healthy subject could also be used to treat an illness with the same characteristics.

Over the following years Hahnemann returned to medical practice, developing the concept of *similia similibus curentur*, by dosing himself, his family and friends with different substances in order to study the symptoms produced when they were given to healthy subjects. These experiments came to be known as *provings*, from the German word *prufung*, meaning 'testing.' This culminated in the publication in 1810 of his book *The Organon of Rational Healing*. In it he set down his developing ideas for his system of homoeopathic medicine.

Initially Hahnemann prescribed his remedies in the standard dosages of the day. However, although his results were good, he found that many of his patients suffered an initial aggravation of their symptoms before receiving the benefit. In an attempt to counter this he started giving one-tenth doses. The results were still good, but the aggravations, though less marked, still occurred. He therefore continued diluting the doses, each time giving a tenth of the previous dose. Predictably the aggravations disappeared, but so too did any beneficial effect. The dilutions had reached a point where there was no more medication present.

Homoeopathy might have died a death at that point had Hahnemann not discovered an incredible phenomenon. He found that by vigorously shaking each progressive dilution, the resultant remedy became not only less likely to produce aggravations, but it became more potent. This process he termed *potentisation.*

Fundamental to his theory of homoeopathy was the concept of the Vital Force. In his view the remedy acted not upon the disease, but upon the Vital Force to restore balance within the body.

Between 1812 and 1821, while he was professor of Medicine at Leipzig, Hahnemann published a six-volume work entitled *The Materia Medica Pura.* It contained the results of all his provings. However, because of a legal wrangle with the apothecaries who tried to sue him on the grounds that he was infringing their right to prepare drugs, he was forced to leave the city and move to Köthen. It was there that he wrote a five-volume work entitled *The Chronic Diseases.* This, together with the Organon and the Materia Medica Pura formed the basis of his homoeopathic theory.

In *The Chronic Diseases* Hahnemann set out to explain why homoeopathy sometimes worked well with acute illnesses, yet failed with chronic disease. He postulated that chronic diseases were due to one of three *miasms,* which he termed *psoric, sycotic and syphilitic.* He believed that they were disturbances in the Vital Force which permeates the body. Sometimes these miasms could be acquired and sometimes they were inherited, thereby exerting an effect through several generations, like 'ghosts of the original illness.'

The spread of homoeopathy

By the time of Hahnemann's death at the age of 88 in 1843, homoeopathy had spread far and wide. In England, Dr Harvey Quin founded the British Homoeopathic Society in 1844 and was instrumental in opening the London Homoeopathic Hospital in 1850.

Other converts to the method carried it further afield. By the end of the nineteenth century there were homoeopathic hospitals all over Europe, Russia, the two Americas and the Indian subcontinent. Indeed, at the present time there are probably more homoeopathic practitioners in India than in any other country in the world.

Dr James Tyler Kent

In the USA, sometime in the mid 1870s a young orthodox-trained physician by the name of James T. Kent called upon the services of a homoeopathic doctor to tend to his ill wife. Standard orthodox treatment had failed to help her and, at her request, she had begged him to try the new medicine. To Kent's surprise a dramatic cure was achieved. From then on Dr Kent determined to find out more about this amazing method. It proved to be a fortuitous day for the development of homoeopathy.

Hahnemann and his helpers had proved around 130 remedies, but over the few years since his death the number had swollen considerably. However, although the body of knowledge had grown, it remained fairly disorganised. That is where Kent proved his worth. He systematised the materia medica to give a clearer picture of each remedy, and he compiled his *Repertory of the Homoeopathic Materia Medica*.

Essentially, the repertory is a book containing every conceivable symptom and the manner in which it is perceived by the individual, or modified by external agents such as temperature, weather, movement etc. It is organised into logical sections and is cross-indexed against all of the appropriate remedies.

Kent's Repertory is one of the main reference works used today by homoeopaths all over the world.

Dr Edward Bach

The last great name I propose to talk about is Dr Edward Bach, the founder of the wonderful system of treatment which bears his name—*the Bach Flower Remedies*.

In the 1920s Dr Edward Bach practised as a pathologist at the London Homoeopathic Hospital and as a homoeopathic physician in Harley Street. In that time he produced a stream of scientific papers and worked with Dr John Patterson in the development of the *bowel nosodes*, a group of remedies which can only really be described as 'homoeopathic vaccines.' For this work he was acclaimed by his colleagues as 'the second Hahnemann.'

Bach's real aim in life was to produce the simplest form of medicine possible, which could be taken by the sufferer him or herself without fear of harm. In 1930, with this in mind he threw up his practice and moved to the country.

He believed that certain negative states of mind resulted in illness, and that by correcting the emotional imbalances a whole-person cure could be obtained. He sought and found these remedies among the flowers of the fields and hedgerows of the English countryside.

Initially, he found twelve plants which were capable of correcting twelve corresponding negative states of mind. His findings were duly written up in his books *Heal Thyself* and the world famous *The Twelve Healers*.

In the years between 1933 and his death in 1936 he found another 26 remedies, to complete the 38 remedies which literally cover all of the negative states of mind that can afflict mankind.

The principles of homoeopathy

From the brief historical outline I have just given it should be fairly clear that the two main principles are the Law of Similars and the use of potentised remedies. Let us now look at them in a little more detail.

THE LAW OF SIMILARS

This means that a substance which produces symptoms of a disease in a well person can also be used to treat someone who has that disease. Hence, *similia similibus curentur*—let like be treated by like.

Effectively one takes the symptom-complex of the patient and attempts to match it up with the toxic effect-complex of a remedy. There may be several remedies which are close, but the nearest match is the 'similar.' As an example, belladonna poisoning causes a toxic effect-complex which resembles the disease of scarlet fever. If someone suffering with scarlet fever presents in the classic manner, then belladonna would be the appropriate similar.

This is a fairly clear cut case. It is important to appreciate, however, that in homoeopathy one is trying to match the remedy profile to the patient profile, not to the disease-profile. To explain this, consider five men all of whom have arthritis affecting the hips. The same orthodox treatment may be appropriate for all five. A homoeopath, however, would look at the symptom patterns of each individual and could well end up prescribing a completely different remedy for each man. It is, after all, the individual that is being treated in homoeopathy and not the disease.

THE LAW OF CURE

One of the main homoeopathic principles is the Law of Cure, formulated by an American homoeopath, Constantine Hering. It states that a cure is affected:

from above downwards
from within outwards
from major to lesser organs
and it takes place in reverse order of appearance of the symptoms.

Thus, one starts to feel emotionally better before the physical improvement comes. Similarly, with an illness which presented with a cough then a rash, the rash (being last to come) would disappear before the cough settled.

REMEDIES FROM MANY SOURCES

The modern homoeopathic materia medica contains well over two thousand remedies. All sorts of things are used, from simple substances like common salt, to exotic cacti, snake venom and precious minerals like gold.

For homoeopathy to be successful one must select the correct remedy. This means that the match between the remedy profile and the patient's symptom profile must be as good as possible. Sometimes the decision is obvious and sometimes it is extremely difficult. There are, you see, many different schools of thought in homoeopathy about what the aim should be with a remedy, how it should be given, at what potency and how often.

The approach used in this book is, I believe, the simplest to understand. We will be focusing upon two types of remedy. Firstly, there is the *constitutional remedy*, which is deep-acting and is appropriate for a patient who conforms to a set type. There may be a particular appearance, pattern of thought, attitude and response to illnesses. Taking one's constitutional remedy is often a way of strengthening oneself and acting on the illness at its very roots.

Secondly, there is the *local remedy*, which acts more superficially and is used to treat particular patterns of illness. For example if we look at a number of people suffering from sciatica, we look at the key features which distinguish their experience and perception of the 'disease' and prescribe accordingly. Although the same condition is being treated, there are at least a dozen remedies which could be used depending upon the key features.

POTENCY AND THE INFINITESIMAL DOSE

Although homoeopathy is associated with using infinitesimal amounts of substances, it is the law of similars which is the crux of the method. If the incorrect remedy is chosen the question of potency is almost irrelevant.

Potency means far more than dilution. The process of potentisation actually seems to enhance the 'power' of a remedy, so that it becomes more potent. The remedy becomes less concentrated but more energised.

In order to prepare homoeopathic medicines two methods are used. Firstly, for soluble substances an alcoholic extract is made by infusion for up to three weeks, followed by filtration to produce a *mother tincture*. This is then diluted with 40 per cent alcohol to one in ten or one in a hundred. Next it is vigorously vibrated for a few seconds, a process called *succussion*, to produce the first potency remedy on the two commonest potency scales.

The 1:10 scale is called the *Decimal scale* and is designated by the letter 'x' in the UK, and by 'D' on the continent. Thus the first potency would be 1x.

The 1:100 scale is called the *Centesimal scale* and is designated by the letter 'c' in the UK, and by 'CH' on the continent. Thus the first potency would be 1c.

To prepare the next potency one part of the first potency would be taken and diluted 1:10 or 1:100, then successed as before to produce the 2x or 2c potencies.

It will by now be very clear that it does not take many dilutions to dramatically reduce the concentration of a substance. By the 6th process on the decimal scale (6x), which is the equivalent of the 3rd on the centesimal scale (3c) the mother tincture will be diluted to one in a million. By the 6th process on the centesimal scale (6c) the dilution will be one in a billion, while by the 30th process (30c) the dilution will be one in five billion. These figures are quite incredible. Indeed, according to Avogadro's Law, by the time one reaches 12c the solution is unlikely to have even a single molecule of the original compound left.

The second method is for insoluble substances which cannot be made into mother tinctures. In this case they are mechanically ground together with lactose powder for several hours in the proportion of one in ten, a process called *trituration*. This process is repeated three times to produce a 3x potency, after which it can be dissolved in alcohol and water and potentised in the usual manner.

By convention 12c is the cut off point, all remedies up to this being considered low potency and those of 12c and above being high potency.

Which potency to use?

Within the world of homoeopathy there is considerable debate as to whether it is best to use low or high potency. Hahnemann himself advocated using the 30th, while Kent would never use anything below 30c. Indeed, he tended to use far higher ones, even going up to the millionth on the centesimal scale. On the other hand many modern European homoeopaths use mixtures of low potency remedies.

Again, since the important thing is the particular remedy selected we need not get too bogged down in the question of potencies. Throughout the book we shall use only two: 6c for low potency treatment and 30c for high potency work.

How do the remedies work?

From what we have just seen about potencies it is clear that only the low potencies can possibly work in the accepted pharmacological sense through a chemical reaction. Once one exceeds Avogadro's number, which happens at 12c, there cannot logically be any of the original remedy left in the solution. If the remedies still work, which they decidedly do, then they clearly must be working in some other more subtle manner. Rather than working biochemically I believe that they are working biophysically.

Research carried out over the past forty or so years has looked at the potency question. Studies on enzymes, the growth of yeasts and seedlings have all demonstrated that appropriate homoeopathic preparations exert an effect even when one has gone past the Avogadro level of 12c.

Curiously, however, it is an observed phenomenon that the effect under study seems to wax and wane with succeeding potency levels. For example, when measuring the effect of a homoeopathic substance on the growth of wheat seedlings a boosting effect may appear at 7c, followed by a retarding effect at 9c, then a boosting effect at 11c. The actual amount of boost received may be no more at 11c than at 7c, as indeed the retarding effect may be the same at 9c, 13c and 17c. This suggests that they are working in an energetic or wave-form manner.

One of the most celebrated pieces of research in recent years was that published by Professor Jaques Benveniste of Paris, in the scientific journal *Nature* in June 1988. He reported upon the ability of 'homoeopathically prepared' (my parentheses) dilutions of Anti-IgE in the range up to 60c to cause particular types of white blood cell to lose their staining ability. Like previous workers he discovered a wave-like effect of activity and inactivity with successive potentisations.

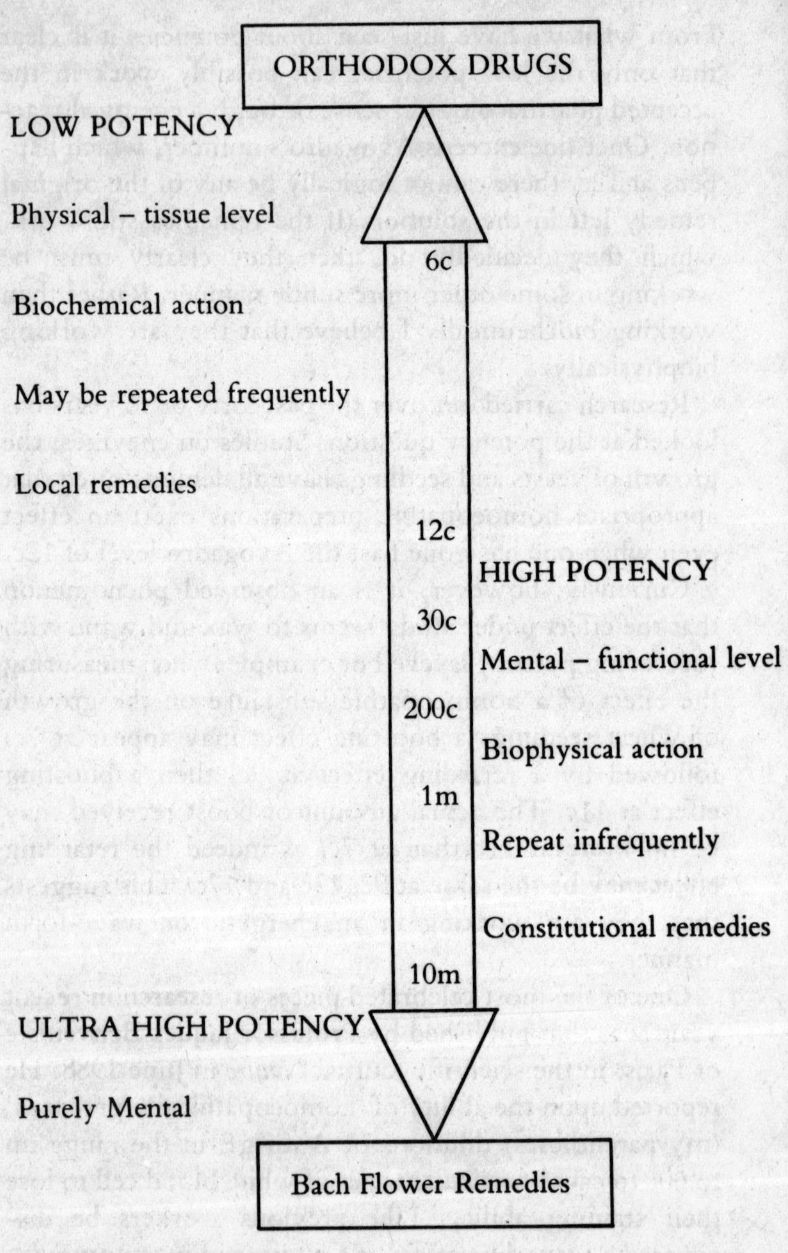
ORTHODOX DRUGS
LOW POTENCY
Physical – tissue level
6c
Biochemical action
May be repeated frequently
Local remedies
12c
HIGH POTENCY
30c
Mental – functional level
200c
Biophysical action
1m
Repeat infrequently
Constitutional remedies
10m
ULTRA HIGH POTENCY
Purely Mental
Bach Flower Remedies

Figure 3

These studies were repeated and confirmed in five other laboratories throughout the world—another in France, two in Israel, one in Italy and one in Canada.

One of Benveniste's conclusions was that since dilutions need to be accompanied by vigorous shaking for the effects to be observed, transmission of the biological information could be related to the molecular organisation of the water. In other words, the water somehow retains an energetic imprint of the original molecule's energy, perhaps retained in the way molecules of water connect to one another through their hydrogen bonding.

And this brings us back to the nature of the remedy itself. It is not the chemistry of the compound used to make the remedy that matters, but its very energy, its *vibrational pattern*. It is the fact that it 'vibrates' in the similar manner to the 'vibration' of the individual's illness, or to the pattern he presents to the world through his symptoms, signs, feelings and attitudes. When he takes the remedy, it is the remedy's vibration which stimulates the etheric body to reharmonise itself, resulting in the ultimate rebalancing of the physical body.

So finally, let me reconsider the potency question. It is my personal opinion that with problems which are most obviously rooted in the physical body the low potencies are more appropriate, since they have more of a biochemical, tissue level effect. On the other hand, where a problem is more 'functional' and associated with emotional symptoms, there is more need to aim the treatment at the etheric body. Thus, since there is more of a need to work at the biophysical range, one should use the higher potencies. Finally, when dealing purely with the emotional side of things one can consider using the Bach Flower Remedies, which though not technically 'homoeopathic' seem to work like ultra-high potency remedies (Figure 3).

4

Types of Constitutions

Study the patient not the disease

James Tyler Kent

As we saw in the last chapter we can use both constitutional and local remedies. Before we examine them in more detail, let's look at the concept of constitutions first.

Throughout history it has been a basic aim of many medical systems to identify 'types' of people. In particular, the desire has been to link up physical characteristics, emotional profiles, strengths and weaknesses in order to work out in what way the individual's internal balance is impaired so that the treatment can be tailored to meet his needs.

According to Ayurvedic Medicine, which is practised extensively throughout India, there are three humours, or vital energies or fluids, which can join together in various combinations at a person's birth. These combinations result in the production of seven constitutional types. Essentially, the Ayurvedic physician aims to determine the individual constitution and treat it appropriately.

Islamic Medicine, which is based upon the teachings of Hippocrates and Galen, also has a humoral theory. Like Ayurveda it proposes that the humours combine together at birth to form a basic constitutional type. And since there are four humours in this system the number of constitutional types is extended to eleven.

The constitution in homoeopathy

In homoeopathy we recognise the concept of the constitutional type. By this we mean the combination of physical and psychological features of the person, together with the way they interact with and react to their environment.

These constitutional types are described in terms of the remedy profile which most closely suits the personality and overall profile of that individual. Thus a homoeopath might talk about an 'Arsenicum type' or a 'Phosphorus' or a 'Sulphur type.'

One thing should be made clear, however, and that is that there are very many different constitutional types of remedies, since each person is an individual. In homoeopathy we make no attempt to categorise people into a set number of categories, as is done in Ayurvedic Medicine and in Unani Medicine. Simply, we try to match up the person profile to the remedy profile.

The constitution and illness

Most homoeopathic remedies have been found to have a range of action in certain disease states. So too, it has been found that different constitutional types have a tendency towards some illnesses. Indeed, some homoeopaths would say that the individual's constitution is programmed to make the individual susceptible to certain diseases. Further than that, some would actually say that there is only *fundamental disease*, which affects the etheric body in a particular manner, making it manifest the disease states at different points in the person's life.

This does not mean that all infections, accidental injuries and psychological traumas are part of the pre-programming of the individual. Of course not. They represent acute problems which affect the individual 'locally.'

By 'fundamental disease,' the concept is being put forward that for some reason or another the 'vibration' of the Vital Force in the etheric body starts to manifest itself as an imbalance. This may exert its effect through the *subtle anatomy and subtle physiology* of the etheric body to produce the effect upon the physical body. This physical illness may then be modified by the environment, by the use of drugs or by apparent 'healing' and burning out of the disease. The body seems to cope and life goes on.

What may be happening, however, is that the fundamental disease effectively stutters on, walling off each episode of what may seem to be unrelated illnesses, until the point is reached where the final 'chronic illness' rears its ugly head—then stays forever, defying any treatment.

The model of chronic disease is thus proposed that fundamental illness starting in early life can be dealt with readily, without producing any structural damage. If, however, the illness is merely suppressed, for example by repeated courses of antibiotics not allowing the body's own defences to cope with the infection, then the illness gets 'walled off' like the layers of a pearl or of an onion. Yet the walling off is not the end of the matter, it merely allows a different vibration which will produce more manifestations later on. The same process may follow until more and more layers are added.

This then is the model of chronic disease. Depending upon the constitutional type it may have manifested itself as a chronic catarrhal problem, a growth problem, a colitis picture, migraine, or anything else which is apt to become chronic or recurrent.

Study the patient not the disease

All orthodox doctors take a case history and take note of the past medical history. Taking note may be all that is done, however, since past 'burned out' conditions are often not thought to be of much significance. To the homoeopath all such things are of potential importance.

They may indicate alterations which need to be made in treatment.

If we accept the model which I have just given, then it should be pretty clear that chronic disease can be very difficult to treat. For example, the use of more and more powerful analgesics and anti-inflammatory agents in arthritis is likely at best to damp down the condition not improve it. With homoeopathy we would have at least two options.

Constitutional or local prescribing

Firstly, we could try to treat constitutionally. This necessitates arriving at the very best match of the patient-profile to a remedy-profile to get the appropriate constitutional remedy. To the classical homoeopath this would be a *deep-acting* high potency remedy which would act directly upon the fundamental disease to get the etheric body to restore harmony throughout the whole person. Such an approach may take a long time, be associated with recurrences of old illnesses and provoke aggravations of the present 'chronic illness.' It may even need more than one type of constitutional remedy.

Such constitutional prescribing is the sort favoured by the Indian and Greek schools of thought.

The second approach would be to use low potency, *superficially-acting* local remedies to act upon the most recent aspects of the illness history. Effectively, therefore, one would be trying to peal back the layers one at a time before focusing on the background state. This is the form of prescribing most favoured by homoeopaths in France and South America.

Aggravation of symptoms

Homoeopathic remedies often produce a temporary aggravation of symptoms as they start to work. When using them in acute conditions the aggravation is usually short-lived, whereas in a more chronic condition it may last for a day or two. Following this one usually finds that the condition starts to improve.

In addition to this, an appropriately chosen constitutional remedy may provoke a *healing crisis* a week or two after taking it. Here the condition seems to worsen and the symptoms of a cold, or tummy bug may seem to come on. Again, this should only last a day or two.

Any new symptoms, such as chest pain, severe abdominal pain, or the passage of blood anywhere is UNLIKELY TO BE DUE TO THE HOMOEOPATHIC REMEDY, SO MEDICAL ADVICE SHOULD BE SOUGHT PROMPTLY.

Selecting a constitutional remedy

There are many more constitutional types in homoeopathy than in any other medical system. This is because everyone is an individual and homoeopathy is the art of bringing medicine to the individual. This being the case, it should be fairly clear that there may be hundreds of constitutional types. If you are able to pin down your own constitutional type then you are fortunate indeed. That remedy can be used for general strengthening and to help the etheric body try to deal with any chronic illness you suffer from.

A CONSTITUTIONAL REMEDY CAN BE TAKEN IN 30c POTENCY AT THE START OF AN ACUTE ILLNESS, OR ONCE A MONTH WHEN DEALING WITH A CHRONIC PROBLEM. (SEE NOTE ON POTENCY AT THE START OF PART THREE)

The main characteristics of an individual are called his or her *generals*. This includes all the things that make you, 'you.' This includes features of importance from the past history, the outlook on life, the reaction to things, etc.

There is a gradation of importance within the generals, these being the following categories:

the mentals—the emotional make-up; psychological tendencies; whether worse or better for such things as consolation, music, stress; introversion or extroversion; fears; sex drive etc.

the modalities—these things or factors which make the individual feel better or worse: being indoors or outdoors; weather preferences; times of the day; preference for movement;

likes and dislikes—foods and drinks; cravings.

disease tendencies—the conditions which this type is prone to. These may have been problems in the past, but have been 'burned out.'

physical features—certain physical features, outlooks and manners may be very relevant.

In addition to the above 'generals' each remedy has '**particulars**,' or certain symptoms which are characteristic.

At this point it is worth having a look through the materia medica in Part Three of the book. This contains the remedy profiles of 57 remedies which are of value in the Third Age. Those which are marked with asterisks are some of the commonest constitutional types. The others are more likely to be of value as local remedies for dealing with specific problems such as may be found in the Therapeutic Index at the end of the book.

LOCAL REMEDIES CAN BE TAKEN AT 6c POTENCY ON A DAILY BASIS. (SEE NOTE ON POTENCY AT THE START OF PART THREE)

Do not be concerned if you cannot find a constitutional match. As I said, the constitutional typing can be very difficult and limitations of space do not permit a more exhaustive index. One thing is important, however, and that is that you should not try to make yourself fit into any of the constitutional types. Unless the match is very good, the remedy is unlikely to work. Quite simply if you cannot see your constitutional type it is probably because it is not present. If that is the case then it may be worth seeing a professional homoeopath for their assessment. This is not necessary, however, if your only need is to deal with local problems as listed in the Therapeutic Index at the end of this book.

Finally, where reference is made to hair colouring, body build and other similar features, these obviously relate to the colouring you had before hair loss or greying altered your appearance. Unless, of course, the changes took place prematurely, in which case the change may be of significance.

5

Catering for Individual Needs

This chapter heading is one of the very cornerstones of homoeopathy. It sums up the observation that what is good for one person can be positively harmful for others. If it is not within your constitution to like something, or to react to it in a beneficial manner, then you may be as well simply avoiding it.

Let's look at three contrasting constitutional remedies.

Calcarea Carbonica

This constitutional type seems to go through definite phases, or potential problem periods as they get older. Looking at the overall picture, however, should give one some insight into the needs of this type of person.

The Calcarea carbonica individual tends to be flabby, easily moved to depression and with generalised slowness of thought and movement.

As a toddler they are slow to produce teeth, but the gums get raw, swollen and painful as the arrival is awaited. With each tooth they seem to get 'teething problems.' They get teething coughs, rashes and bouts of vomiting sour milk.

As they get a bit older they get podgy and like to be left alone. You can sit the Calc carb toddler down and he will not charge around, he will sit, and watch and wait.

In adulthood the podginess may go, yet there will still be a flabby appearance to the face, the neck perhaps seeming slightly thin in proportion. More usually though, the appearance is of a fair, fat, flabby type of person. The handgrip is loose, the energy is low. She will tend to perspire, mainly over the head and chest, even when it isn't hot. She will tire quickly, complain of breathlessness on slight exertion and may get bloating in the abdomen.

Anaemia, gall stones, period problems, warts, cramps of all sorts and swelling of the glands with any infection. All this is she prone to.

In middle age we find the tendency to develop chronic catarrh and chest problems.

In the Third Age the above problems are compounded by all sorts of congestion, including congestive heart failure, chronic obstructive airways disease and chronic constipation. Added to this is the tendency to develop back pains, again reflecting the problem with calcification in the supporting tissue of the body.

And there are fears. All sorts of fears, from impending doom, to developing insanity and even death.

All types of exertion, be it mental or physical, tend to exhaust Calc carb types. This does not mean that they cannot cope, they assuredly can, but it may be at a price. In general they hate the open air, dislike outdoor pursuits and get 'chilled' quite easily.

Early in life they generally love eggs above all other foods, although they are partial to ice cream, sweets, raw vegetables and 'curious tastes' like chalky mixtures. Milk, on the other hand makes them worse. It disagrees with them, from the vomiting of sour milk as a baby to the nausea of milk and milk products advised for the flatulence of adulthood.

Arsenicum album

This type is completely different from Calc carb. These individuals are quick, restless, neat and extremely tidy.

As children they stand out because they are so neat. While other children throw things all around them, leaving rooms in disorder, the Arsenicum album types carefully fold, stack and put away in order. They dislike being dirty and will insist upon being clean. Even the baby unable to talk will let it be known that they are not prepared to sit in a damp or soiled nappy.

As they get a little bit older their sense of aesthetics develops. They like pretty and beautiful things which they can collect, organise and categorise. Unlike Calc carb types, they have the energy to do this. But they are fussy and nervous. This gets more so the older they get. They fuss, bother and worry about other people. They organise the family, organise doctor's appointments and dislike it if someone fails to heed their efforts.

They are neat beyond belief. They feel that everything has a place and they ensure that there is a place for everything. The house often has to be cleaned every day. Dusting must not be skimped on, and everything should be put back where it came from.

They are over-sensitive in every way. Any illness seems the worst it could possibly be. Any pain really 'burns.' Surprisingly, rather than being helped by coolness, the burning pain is improved by heat and warmth.

They absolutely hate the smell of tobacco. They dislike strong smells, strong tastes and bright light. Indeed, darkness may cause distress not just because of the lack of light, but because of what they fear might be lurking there. They will always sleep well wrapped up, without even a toe protruding from the covers, although the head must never be covered.

The fears are a point of contact with Calcarea carbonica, yet the fears are more likely to be verbalised. They will produce palpitations and may stimulate the bowels to be loose.

Loose runny colds, loose diarrhoea and vomiting, loose coughs and asthma, these are illnesses which characterise Arsenicum, as opposed to the congestive picture of

Calcarea carbonica. Problems do also seem to recur 'periodically,' which is, of course, in keeping with their neat, ordered constitutions.

On the other hand, they often do get constipated, but fruit and vegetables curiously often make them worse. They get thirsty, but not for large drinks, preferring to drink small quantities frequently. And fat, seemingly out of character with their fastidiousness and relative dainty habits, is a great favourite.

Phosphorus

This type can be likened to a match. They tend to be tall, slim, delicate-featured, and may have a coppery tinge to the hair. They are usually intelligent, artistic, sensitive and sometimes even clairvoyant.

As a child they are warm, affectionate and gullible. They seem to have boundless energy, then clap out when they are tired. When that happens they want to be quiet, yet they want people about them.

As they get older the artistic tendencies come out. They become more sensitive. They sense atmospheres, they dislike noise and they get a 'feeling' when introduced to people. They warm to them or 'tune' into their wavelengths so that they get the feeling of knowing them. They may feel that they can predict what they are going to say.

They tend to fidget and they can be quite impatient. Like a match bursting into flame, they fly into a sudden temper. And, like a match, it is soon burned out and they feel sorry.

They get anxious about things. They often don't understand why, it is just a feeling of dread that comes over them, as if they are responding to an atmosphere.

Their circulation proves an embarrassment to them. In company they can blush profoundly. Indeed, any excitement produces a flare of colour, like the match again.

In general they dislike the damp, although they do

prefer to be out of doors. Sports are enjoyed, but they tend to be fair-weather sports people, who tire easily.

Exercise often causes them to feel stiff, but it is a stiffness which responds to massage. They like this contact.

Tiredness means they need sleep. However, the sleep may be very restless. They tend to start during their sleep and they experience nightmares. Upon waking they feel that they could have had more sleep, yet they notice that other conditions improve with the sleep.

Salt is one of their cravings. They love salty, spicey foods and prefer their drinks to be cold. Indeed, a stomach upset tends to burn (like the match again) and settles with a cold drink, only to cause retching after it has warmed up in the stomach. Generally though, symptoms improve after eating.

Irritation of membranes is common. Winds make the eyes and nose smart and they go red. This irritation also tends to make them prone to all sorts of all haemorrhagic conditions. For example, nose bleeds come quickly after a flare up of emotion or anger. They suffer from piles, blood in the urine and sometimes colitis. Menstrual problems are common.

The respiratory tract is also a weakness. They suffer from coughs, asthma, and pneumonia. Often they feel worse lying on their backs or on the affected side.

Too long in bed tends to cause breakdown of tissue. Thus bed sores and thrombophlebitis are common in the Third Age.

From the above three constitutional pictures it is clear that these types have very different traits. Calcarea carbonica types love eggs, raw vegetables and sweets, but are made worse by milk. Arsenicum album like fats and milk, sometimes like sweets, but may be upset by ice cream, raw fruits and vegetables. Phosphorus likes salt and spices, feels better for eating, but only prefers cold drinks. Arsenicum album also likes cold drinks, but the reason there is that they don't like their mouths to go dry, rather than because they are thirsty.

Physical and mental exercise makes Calcarea types worse. Arsenicum likes mental work, but copes with physical activities which are well-regulated. Not for them a free for all or a jam session. On the other hand, Phosphorus quite likes being in the limelight, as long as the conditions are right.

Some cases

These are just some examples of the ways in which different constitutions have different cravings, different reactions and different needs. But so far we have been talking in generalities. Let's now look at some cases.

Mrs S.C., aged 63, widowed at the age of 61. After her bereavement she developed thundering headaches and was found to have high blood pressure. She was put on antihypertensive medication and a salt-free diet. She struggled with the diet, found herself craving cheese, crisps, smoked fish and other high-salt foods. The headaches increased in intensity and she became more depressed and started to suffer from back pain.

She was diagnosed as Natrum muriaticum, a classic salt-craver. Allowing her to resume her normal diet immediately lessened the severity of the headaches, improved the back pain and the depression. The blood pressure was not adversely affected by the salt in the diet, so the antihypertensive medication was left unchanged.

Treatment with high potency Natrum Muriaticum cleared up the rest of the headaches.

Mr R.J., aged 72, a retired solicitor had a heart attack following an operation for the removal of a warty growth inside his bladder. After discharge home he started to suffer from drop attacks and palpitations. He was readmitted to hospital, put on various medicines and put on a strict diet excluding tea, coffee and told to stop smoking his cigars.

Although the heart problem improved he became very irritable, he developed warts on his hands and his nose. He resented the reduction in his tea consumption, which amounted to ten cups a day.

He was diagnosed as Thuja occidentalis. He was allowed his tea, which made no difference to the heart condition, and he was treated with Thuja in high potency. His irritability improved, as did the warts, quite spontaneously over the following six weeks.

Mr E.P., aged 57, a clerical worker. At a routine medical examination he was found to have an archus senilus, a ring of white discolouration just inside the rim of his irises. This is sometimes associated with a raised blood fat level. Accordingly, a blood test was performed, which confirmed a raised cholesterol level. He was advised to reduce his fat intake and take gentle exercise.

Within weeks he started to complain of anxiety, irritability, strange piercing pains in his throat and in his rectum. Haemorrhoids were found on examination, which did not respond to soothing creams and suppositories.

He was diagnosed as Nitricum acidum, the fat restriction was rescinded and his symptoms improved, clearing up after treatment with the remedy in high potency.

Miss L.W., aged 88, a retired nurse. She had been fairly independent until the age of 80, when she moved into a nursing home. She liked to keep herself to herself, was anxious about meeting people, yet always seemed fairly cheerful. She was proud and neat, so it mortified her when she began to be incontinent at night. She started to get cantankerous.

Sleep had always been a problem to her, so she tended to take cat-naps throughout the day. The staff at the nursing home tried to get her into a regular sleep routine, the idea being to stop the cat-naps and get her to sleep right through, having been taken to the toilet last thing at night. Her problem with incontinence became worse as did her cantankerousness.

She was diagnosed as Causticum. She was allowed to sleep when she wanted and was given Causticum, with improvement in mood, incontinence and sleep cycle.

Mrs T.T., aged 72, slipped and fell on the ice, breaking her left hip. After the operation to repair it, as she was forced to rest, she became very depressed, lacking in energy and basically withdrew from her family. Nothing they did seemed to help her. Indeed, much to the daughter's distress, she became indifferent to everyone, especially her husband who was looking after her despite a heart complaint.

Up until the accident she had apparently always enjoyed bowling and dancing. Her enforced rest had affected her badly and she was encouraged to become active as quickly as possible. The first trip to the bowling club brought a swift, if short-lived, improvement in her spirits and attitude. She was diagnosed as Sepia and prescribed accordingly. Her improvement was welcomed by the whole family.

Eat a balanced diet but respect the constitution

From the above cases it should be clear that people have differing needs. Forcing yourself to eat a particularly restrictive diet may mean eating outwith your constitutional desires. This does not mean that you should be faddist about your food, but that you should try to eat a balanced diet, making allowances for your constitution. In other words, if it is part of your nature to crave a foodstuff, don't completely exclude it. Similarly, if you have a particular aversion to a group of foodstuffs, don't make them a major part of your diet—if at all. There are always alternatives. Remember, eating should be enjoyable. Let's look at a few examples.

SALT

People are put onto salt-free diets for all sorts of spurious reasons. It may be because of water retention, high blood pressure or leg ulcerations. Stopping added salt may merely heighten the craving for high-salt foods, such as canned or smoked meats and fish, cheese, soups, yeast extracts, crisps and savouries. Eliminating everything may upset the whole balance, as in the first individual case mentioned earlier.

(Natrum muriaticum, Nitricum acidum and Phosphorus all love salt.)

MILK AND DAIRY PRODUCTS

Milk diets have traditionally been given for people suffering from peptic ulcers. Many antacid preparations are also made from milk products. The milk hater may worsen from the addition of it to the diet.

(Natrum carbonicum and Lac defloratum hate milk. It disagrees with Calc carb and Phosphorus may be upset by boiled milk drinks.)

FATS

China, Petroleum and Pulsatilla all hate fat, while Arsenicum album, Hepar sulph, Nitric acidum, Nux vomica and Sulphur all enjoy it. Care should be taken in excluding it completely from the diets of the constitutional fat-likers.

A balanced diet in the Third Age

In the Third Age there is a need to have a healthy diet. What exactly this should be, however, has never been very clear. In 1965 the King Edward's Hospital Fund report of an investigation into the diet of elderly women living alone, stated, 'the precise nutritional needs of old people are unknown.' Quarter of a century later the state of knowledge is still misty.

I do not think it is possible to say that there is an ideal diet for people in the Third Age. We are, after all, talking about a group ranging from the very fit and active to the frail and infirm. In my opinion the three main aims of diet are to:

avoid obesity
avoid deficiency states
avoid constipation

A 'balanced diet' should contain an adequate amount of all essential nutrients plus sufficient fibre to prevent constipation. It should of course be appreciated that since the energy expenditure tends to drop in the Third Age, mainly because we become less active and less energetic, you have to take care not to exceed the energy requirements, otherwise you become obese.

PROTEIN

It is important to take in adequate amounts of protein from foods such as lean meat, eggs, dairy products, beans, soya, corn and peas. A portion of lean meat or poultry a day, on most days would be acceptable. Three to four eggs should be the maximum per week.

Soya, lentils and other 'sprouts' are particularly recommended for women in the Third Age, because they are rich in phyto-oestrogens. These may help menopausal and post-menopausal problems. (See Chapter 14.)

FAT

Despite all the calls for avoiding fat in the diet, some fat is necessary. Indeed, in the Third Age this is important, otherwise a deficiency of one of the fat-soluble vitamins can occur. These include: Vitamin A, which is essential for the maintenance of mucous membranes in the eyes, ears, nose, throat, lungs and bladder; Vitamin D, which is essential for calcium absorption and hence for the state of the skeleton; Vitamin E, an antioxidant, vital for maintaining the integrity of cell membranes; and Vitamin K, necessary for the clotting mechanism of the blood.

Fatty fish, such as salmon, trout, mackerel and sardines are excellent sources of fat and of the fat soluble Vitamin D. A portion at least twice a week would be beneficial. Extra Virgin Olive Oil is also an extremely good source, added to salads.

CARBOHYDRATES

These are high energy foods. It is probably as well to restrict sugars and try to take the bulk of carbohydrates in unrefined, high fibre form. For example, beans, lentils, all vegetables and wholemeal bread. These are excellent for preventing constipation and should be eaten freely.

ANTIOXIDANTS

I mentioned about the Free Radical Theory in Chapter One. To recap, it is thought that in all sorts of metabolic processes there is a release of molecules with unpaired electrons. These 'free radicals' are thought to promote oxidation which can damage DNA, cell membranes, enzymes, proteins and fat molecules. Effectively, it is a process similar to the rotting of an elastic band.

The older one becomes the more is this thought to happen, with consequently more damage to cells and biological structures throughout the body.

It is also thought that some protection is offered against the free radical reactions by 'antioxidants.' Natural antioxidants are: Vitamin E, carotene (the name for a group of substances which can be converted by the body into Vitamin A), various enzymes and Vitamin C. The main source for these are nuts, fruit and vegetables, especially raw ones. Particularly rich are many of the foods with a bright orange colour, such as carrots, apricots, pumpkin and cantaloup melon. All of these should be eaten freely. Indeed, a recent study of 34,000 Americans showed that those who ate a handful of nuts (peanuts, almonds or walnuts) five times a week, had half the risk of heart attacks, compared to those who only ate them once a week.

A handful of nuts a day is therefore a good addition to the diet.

Exercise and the Third Age

Just as it is not possible to be dogmatic about diet, it is not possible to say what is the ideal amount of exercise for people in the Third Age. Moderation would seem to be the key.

In a nine year study of men aged 40–59 years, the British Heart Foundation followed up 8,000 men in order to assess whether exercise was useful in reducing the risk of heart attacks and strokes. The conclusion was that moderate exercise (a round of golf a week, gardening at the weekend, or a swim) was beneficial in reducing the risk of both heart attacks and strokes. Vigorous exercise, on the other hand was found to reduce further the risk of having a stroke, but increased the chance of having a heart attack.

In the Third Age, it is important not to do vigorous exercise. One should learn new limits and not go beyond them. But again, it is important to look at the constitution and fit the activity to the individual. Exercise can be harmful to sedentary types, just as it can be problematic to enforce rest upon those who are better for keeping on the move.

PART TWO

Tackling Problems of Middle and Old Age

6

Changing Attitudes

Take no notice of the disease, think only of the outlook on life of the one in distress.

Dr Edward Bach

People vary in their outlook on life. For example, there are optimists and pessimists; brave hearts and shrinking violets; decision-makers and waverers. Sometimes the outlook is inborn and sometimes it is acquired. Whichever is the case, however, the way we feel has much to do with the way we live, age and die.

In Chapter Four I discussed the prime importance of considering the 'mentals,' the mind symptoms, when trying to work out a constitutional remedy. It was from this standpoint that Dr Edward Bach, a highly respected homoeopathic physician and bacteriologist, developed his world famous Flower Remedies in the 1930s.

The germ of the idea came to him in 1928, at a time when he was completing his historic work on the bowel nosodes. While attending a banquet he happened to notice that many of the people present could be placed into different groups according to the way they behaved, ate, talked and used body language. In short, his mind was going through the homoeopathic diagnostic process, although with the intention of classifying people into mental groups rather than into remedy types. It did not take him long to reason that particular types of people tended to suffer from particular negative mental states, and, by extension, that this affected their vitality to produce illness.

So convinced was Edward Bach of the importance of this approach that in 1930 he gave up his practice and devoted the rest of his life to finding the appropriate remedies which could cure these negative mental states. His theory was that by correcting the negative state the vitality would be restored, thereby allowing the body to heal itself.

Your outlook

I have no doubt whatsoever that the way we feel affects our whole being. If you get out of balance then negative mental states creep in. Either they will be the mental states associated with your personality, or they will be transient mental states created by circumstances and conditions in your life.

For example, supposing a man is generally lacking in confidence and is suddenly put in the situation of having to give a public lecture. His general lack of confidence makes him doubtful of his ability to give the lecture. Then as the days go by he finds himself becoming more and more fearful of the whole thing. He is unable to eat or sleep and his mind dwells on the prospective lecture. In this situation the lack of confidence is the personality type and the feeling of fear is the response to the fact that he will have to speak in public.

As we shall see shortly, we could consider giving him *larch* for his lack of confidence, and *mimulus* for his specific fear of speaking in public.

The Third Age is obviously a time when all sorts of life events can spring up at us. Retirement, bereavement, infirmity, isolation—all of them can affect our outlook upon life. They can make us anxious, angry, depressed, impatient, or just unhappy in several other ways. It is these negative states which alter our whole well-being, make us ill and feel old. Edward Bach's method was to concentrate upon that outlook and treat it with the appropriate flower remedy.

The Bach Flower Remedies

Dr Bach discovered 38 remedies, which he classified into the following seven groups according to the emotional states which they could cure:

Fear
Uncertainty
Insufficient interest in present circumstances
Loneliness
Over-sensitiveness to influences and ideas
Despondency or despair
Over-care for the welfare of others

The main indications for the remedies in each group are as follows:

FOR FEAR

Rock Rose An emergency remedy for terror or panic.

Mimulus For shy, timid types. Fear of specific things.

Cherry Plum For fear of loss of reason or control. Fear that could do harm to others.

Aspen For fear of unknown origin.

FOR UNCERTAINTY

Cerato For those who doubt their own judgement. They always have to ask people for their opinions.

Scleranthus For quiet types who keep themselves to themselves. They find making decisions difficult. Their moods fluctuate.

Gentian For those who are easily discouraged and who become dejected and despondent.

Gorse For those who suffer utter despair.

Hornbeam For mental and physical fatigue. For those who procrastinate. For the 'Monday morning feeling.'

Wild Oat For those who are indecisive. Helpful in making plans for the future.

FOR INSUFFICIENT INTEREST IN PRESENT CIRCUMSTANCES

Clematis For dreamy, inattentive people who seem to live in their own world, always dreaming about the future. They are unhappy with their own world and want to escape.

Honeysuckle For those who live in the past.

Wild Rose For those who just 'drift on' without making any effort to find joy, or improve things. They become apathetic.

Olive For those drained of mental and physical energy. Everything becomes an effort.

White Chestnut For those who cannot free themselves of some unwanted thought. It buzzes around in their mind.

Mustard For those who are subject to episodes of gloom. The feeling may fall like a curtain, dropping them into a black depression for no obvious reason.

Chestnut Bud For those who fail to learn by experience.

FOR LONELINESS

Water Violet For very quiet, independent people. They like to be left to themselves. Often very intelligent.

Impatiens For impatience and irritability. They want everything done in a hurry. They do not tolerate slowness in others.

Heather For those who are totally self-interested. They seek any available company, because they hate to be left alone. They will talk to anyone about their own problems.

FOR OVER-SENSITIVENESS TO INFLUENCES AND IDEAS

Agrimony For those who try to remain of cheery appearance, despite enduring considerable inner torture. They may drink too much to help themselves cope.

Centaury For those who find it difficult to say 'no.' They let people ride rough-shod over them. They are timid and weak-willed.

Walnut For those who are bound in the past, family or habits by strong links. For those who need help coming to terms with life changes.

Holly For those who suffer from jealousy, suspicion and anger. For strong negative emotions like 'hate.'

FOR DESPONDENCY OR DESPAIR

Larch For those who lack confidence and always expect to fail.

Pine For those who feel guilt and who blame themselves for everything.

Elm For those who feel overwhelmed by responsibility.

Sweet Chestnut For feelings of anguish, as if the limits of endurance have been passed and only oblivion is left.

Star of Bethlehem For the shock of serious news, fright after an accident, a bereavement, etc.

Willow For those who feel sorry for themselves.

Oak For those who struggle bravely on in the face of adversity, even though everything may seem hopeless. They get cross if illness interferes with their duties or helping others.

Crab Apple The cleansing remedy. For those who feel unclean and are disgusted. They are ashamed of their bodies and their illnesses.

FOR OVER-CARE FOR THE WELFARE OF OTHERS

Chicory For those who tend to be over-possessive. They want others to conform to their standards. They may nag others and make martyrs of themselves. They may feign or exaggerate illness in order to maintain control over others.

Vervain For the fanatical, perfectionist and highly-strung. They are rigid, tend never to change their views and want to convert others to their ways. They are incensed by seeming injustices.

Vine For the ruthless, domineering and tyrannical. They like power and they make or have made good leaders.

Beech For the critical and intolerant types. They tend to be arrogant.

Rock Water For the self-disciplinarians who may be too hard on themselves. They may overwork and deny themselves things if their work is interrupted through 'flippancies.'

THE RESCUE REMEDY

An extremely useful composite remedy was also formulated by Dr Bach, for dealing with the emotional effects of shock from any cause. It consists of Star of Bethlehem for shock; Rock Rose for terror and panic; Impatiens for tension and stress; Cherry Plum for desperation and Clematis for feeling faint.

It is useful for taking during bereavement, for stage fright, after traumas of both physical and mental form, and for all acute shocks.

In my day-to-day work I always carry a bottle of Rescue Remedy in my bag.

Taking the Flower Remedies

Stock bottles of the Bach Flower Remedies can be obtained from many chemists and most health shops. A complete set of all thirty-eight is not necessary, since one can usually identify the individual's personality or temperament type and the sort of outlook they tend to adopt.

For temporary negative mental states 2 drops of the appropriate stock remedy should be taken in a cup of water or fresh fruit juice and sipped. If the correct remedy has been chosen then that may be all that is necessary. On the other hand, you can prepare a small bottle of 30 ml capacity by pouring the 2 drops into the bottle then topping up with natural spring water. The dose is then 4 drops directly onto the tongue, four times a day or as often as is necessary until the negative state disappears.

More than one remedy can be taken at a time in a diluted 30 ml bottle, using up to 6 remedies. However, success is greatest when using the smallest number at a time.

With the Rescue Remedy use 4 drops at a time, both when using it on its own and when adding it to a bottle with other remedies. In the latter case it can be counted as a single remedy.

I find that a cup of the appropriate remedy first thing in the morning after analysing the way one is feeling can work wonders.

THE REMEDIES ARE COMPLETELY SAFE AND THERE IS NO DANGER OF INTERACTIONS WITH DRUGS OR OTHER HOMOEOPATHIC PREPARATIONS.

Situations which may affect the way you feel

There are many situations and events in the Third Age which can create negative mental states. We shall now consider a few of the Bach Remedies and homoeopathic remedies which may be helpful. The homoeopathic remedies may all be given for a few doses in either 6c or 30c potencies.

ACCIDENTS

For dealing with the shock of a personal trauma, either physical or mental, or upon hearing of bad news.

BACH FLOWER REMEDIES *Star of Bethlehem* is excellent after hearing about accidents. *Rescue Remedy* is more multi-purpose. Indeed, it is one to have in the medicine cabinet.

Aconite—after any accident where there is shock and you feel frightened and irritable.

Arnica—after any injury where there is bruising.

Ignatia—after fainting at the sight of blood from an accident. If develop illness after bad news.

BEREAVEMENT

BACH FLOWER REMEDIES Think of *Star of Bethlehem* at the start. Then consider the outlook upon life as one goes through the grieving process. For example there may be anger (*holly*), a tendency to live in the past (*honeysuckle*), depression (*mustard*), guilt (*pine*), and difficulty coming to terms with the bereavement (*walnut*). These are all examples, the outlook needing to be assessed and treated accordingly.

Aurum metallicum—when the grief causes constant thoughts of death and suicide. An illness may be provoked by the grief.

Causticum—when the grief causes other ailments. May be irritable in their own grief, but intensely sympathetic to another's.

Ignatia—where there is an hysterical reaction. When one goes to pieces. Tend to just sit and sigh a lot. Worse for sympathy.

Nat Mur—if the grieving process has gone on for a long time, or if problems started after the bereavement. May be quite touchy. Worse for sympathy. May suffer from hammering headaches.

Pulsatilla—for shy people who are better for sympathy. Very weepy and are made to weep by all reminders, sad music, etc.

MAJOR ILLNESSES

Some people take major illnesses in their stride, others wither away, and others fear for their lives. Consider here the effects of heart attacks, strokes, operations, and any major trauma.

BACH FLOWER REMEDIES There may be terror and panic (*Rock Rose or Rescue Remedy*); fear of the illness or of pain (*mimulus*); despair of getting better (*gorse*); complete exhaustion (*olive*); depression (*mustard*); complete introspection about 'the illness' and 'the problem' (*heather*) and again, difficulty in accepting it (*walnut*).

Aconite—when shocked by the situation and fearful of death.

Arsenicum album—when everything seems to be as bad as possible. When there is extreme restlessness and despair of getting better.

Kali phos—if feels lacking in energy and very tense and nervous.

Pulsatilla—when there is fear of death with floods of tears.

Staphysagria—where there is anger with the illness.

RETIREMENT

The best remedy for retirement is preparation. However, despite the best of intentions some people find it a traumatic time.

BACH FLOWER REMEDIES Again, assess the outlook. Breaking the links (*walnut*) is often necessary, as is determining what to do next (*wild oat*). Some people find decision making difficult (*scleranthus*), while others need to stop feeling sorry for themselves (*willow*). Resentment about no longer being part of the work force is also common (*holly*).

Bryonia—where the main talk is of work and business.

Ferrum metallicum—where one is better for mental exertion.

Sepia—where there is a need to keep busy. One feels indifferent to others and comes alive when occupied physically.

* * *

The Bach Flower Remedies are, in my opinion, well worth studying and getting to know well. They are the mainstay of my therapeutic armamenterium for all sorts of psychological and emotional states. Used judiciously they do make you feel well and—hopefully—stop you from worrying about ageing.

Recommended reading: *The Twelve Healers* by Edward Bach MB, BS, MRCS, LRCP, DPH. Published by The C. W. Daniel Co Ltd. Saffron Walden, Essex.

7

Insomnia

Blessings on him who invented sleep,
the mantle that covers all human thoughts.

Don Quixote (Miguel de Cervantes)

To such a madcap as the worthy Don Quixote the mantle of sleep must indeed have seemed a welcome night-garment. Unfortunately, for the majority of people in the Third Age sleep can prove to be an elusive butterfly.

Normal sleep and insomnia

Research in sleep laboratories has shown that during uninterrupted sleep a young adult drifts through four progressively deeper stages of non-rapid eye movement sleep (NREM sleep), associated with slow wave activity on the electroencephalogram (EEG or brain wave tracing). After about ninety minutes the first episode of rapid eye movement sleep (REM sleep) is entered, when muscle relaxation takes place and dreaming occurs. These REM episodes recur about five times during a sleep of 7–8 hours and occupy about 25 per cent of the total.

However, sleep time is not to be equated with 'good sleep.' While some people awake refreshed after only four or five hours' sleep, some people will not be satisfied unless they have had their 'full eight hours' of unbroken sleep. Insomnia is therefore a subjective complaint.

A reasonable working definition of insomnia could therefore be 'A complaint of difficulty in initiating and/ or maintaining sleep which is satisfying.'

Insomnia in the Third Age

Most people experience sleep difficulties as they get older. For one thing the whole physiology of sleep alters. The amount of 'slow wave' sleep is reduced so that periods of wakefulness increase to cause broken, fragmented and unsatisfying sleep. To compensate for this many people take to having cat-naps, which of course will reduce the need for night-time sleep.

The expectation of sleep is often part of the problem, since people expect to need and get eight hours. The reality, however, is that four to six hours' sleep is the norm and, as long as one does not feel tired upon waking there is no need for more.

Some causes of insomnia

Apart from the normal changes that take place in the sleep cycle with age, most cases of correctable insomnia can be attributed to pain, worry or drugs.

It obviously makes no sense to treat insomnia caused by painful conditions with sedatives or hypnotic medications. Similarly, emotional problems are merely numbed by the use of sleeping pills. And finally, if a drug has sleep disturbance as a side effect, it is clearly an unacceptable drug.

Caffeine in tea and coffee, various breathing tablets, diuretics, anti-depressants and Beta-blockers can all cause insomnia. Indeed, paradoxically so can many hypnotics themselves. The problem is that they tend to reduce REM sleep, thereby eventually causing wakefulness as tolerance increases to the drug.

Self-help measures

It is important that you do not make any alteration in your orthodox medication without first consulting your doctor.

Stop drinking tea or coffee after tea-time is worth doing, possibly going onto a herbal tea such as camomile, peppermint, sage or rose-hip. Herbal tea-bags of all of these are available from most health shops. I find that they are best taken fairly weak, any bitterness being countered by about quarter of an inch worth of cut liquorice root, or a half spoonful of honey.

It is important not to overload the stomach last thing at night. A small snack is acceptable, although cheese and chocolate may keep you awake.

Smoking last thing at night might make you feel relaxed, but it will in fact heighten your wakefulness and delay sleep.

Finally while alcohol is fairly good at inducing sleep, it may well cause broken sleep by reason of its diuretic effect. A little may be useful, but too much is likely to be unhelpful.

Homoeopathic treatment

Bach Flower Remedies

Negative mental states can keep one awake. As always the secret of success with these remedies is in correctly identifying that state. A cup of the appropriate remedy prior to bed, or several times during that day in the usual manner may well solve the problem.

Agrimony—where there is distress, worry and restlessness, although the individual puts on a jolly exterior.

Elm—if one feels pressured and overwhelmed by responsibilities.

Hornbeam—where sleep is unsatisfying because of waking with a Monday morning feeling.

Mimulus—if there is fear of falling asleep and never waking.

Olive—where there is exhaustion so severe that sleep will not come.

White Chestnut—where the mind is in a spin with unwanted thoughts.

Arnica—feels exhausted, but unable to sleep. The bed feels hard.

Arsenicum album—for restlessness and anxiety. Wakes in the early hours. May have periodic upsets in sleep.

Belladonna—if the legs are restless and jerk you awake.

China—if thoughts crowd in at night. Especially if debilitated from diarrhoea, excess perspiration, blood loss, excessive laxative usage.

Coffea—if unable to switch off. Starts awake at the slightest noise.

Ignatia—if there is an unstoppable yearning to yawn repeatedly. Sleep won't come.

Nux Vomica—if there is indigestion after too rich food. May wake in a bad mood.

Phosphorus—if there are nightmares.

Spigelia—if kept awake by palpitations every night.

Sulphur—if tends to talk, grunt, snore in fitful sleep. Tends to stick the limbs outside the bed because they feel hot.

8

Failing Senses

The five senses—sight, hearing, taste, smell and touch—are the means by which we experience the physical world in which we live. The information that they feed into the nervous system is analysed by the brain so that one can perceive whatever is being presented to that particular sense organ.

Age, illness, environmental damage and drugs can all alter the senses. The same applies to the tissue of the brain and, therefore, the function of the mind.

Confusion is relatively common in the Third Age. This can arise from such things as:

depression,
toxic states such as acute infections,
drug side effects,
cerebro-vascular disease,
vitamin and nutritional deficiencies,
hypothyroidism,
dementia.

Sensory loss is also common. While in India the estimates are vague, over 70,000 people over the age of 65 are registered blind in the UK Very many more have a visual problem of one form or another, many of which are correctable or treatable. In addition, probably hundreds of thousands of people over the age of 65 are deaf or hard of hearing. Again, this is probably only the tip of the iceberg, with about ten times that number having some hearing deficit.

Loss of smell is usually due to a catarrhal problem. When this sense is impaired the sense of taste is usually also reduced, because the two are intimately connected.

IT IS ALWAYS WORTH HAVING THE SENSES CHECKED OUT, SINCE A PROBLEM MAY WELL BE CORRECTABLE.

Aluminium—a metal to be wary of

It has been known for many years that aluminium is neurotoxic, or poisonous to nerve tissue. It has also been recorded that there is often an increase in the aluminium content of the brain in senile dementia, or Alzheimer's disease. It is similarly thought to be toxic to the liver, kidneys and bones.

Aluminium can be taken into the body through cooking with aluminium utensils or storing food in aluminium foil. It is also present in some food additives used in processed cheese, baking powder, salt, coffee whiteners and some antacids.

There seems to be a close relationship between calcium, magnesium and aluminium. Deficiency of either of the first two seems to provoke the problems caused by aluminium.

It is advisable for people in the Third Age to avoid the use of aluminium cooking utensils or foil, particularly if there has been any problem with concentration or memory. Similarly, one should ensure that there is sufficient calcium in the diet. (See Chapter 10.) While the aluminium may not be the cause of the problem it might possibly be aggravating it.

MEMORY PROBLEMS

The cause of the memory problem should if possible be diagnosed, so a professional opinion is advisable prior to using any type of medication.

Alumina—for memory which is worse in the morning, but improving as the day goes on. Worth giving if aluminium cooking utensils are used.

Ambra grisea—for memory loss in frail, trembling

people. There is a tendency to flit from one question to another, as if the purpose of the first question is forgotten as the second one comes to mind.

Anacardium orientale—for memory loss associated with irritability, possibly with a tendency to swear. This may be in someone with a fairly strong moral sense, so that they feel guilty about the swearing, yet are unable to stop themselves from doing so.

Apis mellifica—for memory loss, tearfulness, whining and clumsiness.

Baryta carbonica—where there is memory loss, difficulty concentrating and childish behaviour. Thinking about the memory loss or other problems makes matters worse.

Causticum—where the memory is poor, particularly when trying to think. Becomes irritable, yet always sympathetic to other's problems.

Cocculus—where there is general slowness of thought, concentration and memory. Finds trouble getting the right word. Hates contradiction.

Lycopodium—where there is worry that the memory deficit is worse than it is. Wears a worried frown.

Rhododendron—where the thoughts simply disappear. Worse in thunderstorms.

EYE PROBLEMS

Pain in the eye must always be treated seriously, since it could be due to glaucoma or iritis. Both of these conditions, as also cataract, can cause loss of vision, so an urgent medical opinion should be sought. Yet another dangerous condition is temporal arteritis, which is indicated by a fearful thumping headache. Again, a medical opinion should be sought if such a pain starts for the first time ever.

Apis—for pale pink watery swelling of the eyelids, with a burning discomfort.

Euphrasia—for burning discomfort in eyes which water all the time. When there is blurred vision, particularly in the presence of early cataracts.

Gelsemium—when there is dimness of vision and discomfort on moving the eyes.

Phosphorus—when the vision seems misty and it is necessary to shade the eyes. Again, cataracts may be developing.

Ruta—when there is a feeling of dimness of vision after 'straining' the eyes.

HEARING PROBLEMS—DEAFNESS AND TINNITUS

Since hearing problems can become very debilitating (and since some, such as wax, are easily dealt with) it is important to have the ears checked out first.

Causticum—when there is deafness, tinnitus (ringing in the ears) and a sensation of the voice echoing.

China officinalis—when there is deafness, tinnitus and tenderness of the ears in a debilitated person.

Lycopodium—when there is deafness and discharge from the ears. Tends to have a worried frown.

Nitricum acidum—when there is deafness which is better in a noisy room. May get splinter-like discomfort from time to time.

PROBLEMS WITH THE SENSE OF SMELL

Anacardium orientale—for reduced and distorted sense of smell with nasal obstruction. Frequent sneezing.

Calcarea carbonica—for reduced sense of smell with nasal polyps.

Natrum muriaticum—for reduced smell with a cold that starts with sneezing. Usually craves salty things.

Phosphorus—for reduced sense of smell coupled with a burning feeling and a tendency towards nose-bleeds.

Pulsatilla—for reduced sense of smell varying with the amount of catarrh. This varies from day to day and from hour to hour. Worse for stuffy rooms. Prefers the open air.

REDUCED SENSE OF TASTE

This may occur together with alterations in the sense of smell.

Natrum muriaticum—for reduced sense of taste and smell. The nose runs profusely.

Phosphorus—for dry, red tongue and loss of taste. May get nose-bleeds.

Silica—when the taste is reduced and there is the feeling of having a hair in the mouth or on the tongue.

9

Coping with Pain

Pain is one of the commonest complaints, yet is sometimes very difficult to define. The thing is that pain is not an actual entity itself. It is an experience that is unique to the person who is having it. It is this fact that makes homoeopathy a useful approach to its management.

Before going further it is as well to differentiate acute from chronic pain. Many people mistakenly think that they are two poles of a spectrum of experience. This is not the case.

'Acute' pain is the expected physiological response to a stimulation which is immediately perceived as being noxious to the body. The simplest example is the immediate withdrawal reflex of your hand when you burn the fingers. If the burn is mild the pain will go in a relatively short period of time. This type of pain is seen to have a purpose, in that it alerts the body to a problem that it can readily relieve.

'Chronic' pain, on the other hand, is the continual experience of an unpleasant sensation which is unlikely to disappear of its own accord. For example, you can have the chronic pain of arthritis. Unlike acute pain, it should be clear that this type of pain has no useful function. It just grinds away at you and can make life quite miserable. Clearly, coping with chronic pain can be difficult, since it is never easy to ignore pain. Indeed, in some people the intensity can be such that pain dominates their life.

People who experience unrelieved pain over a considerable period of time usually feel trapped and helpless. Often a vicious circle develops which keeps them chained to their pain. For example, after losing sleep for some time it is common to feel *anxious*. This in turn eventually makes them withdraw from friends and relatives, because it is felt that no-one can really understand what they are going through. The result is that they experience *isolation*. Finally, because they feel isolated, they spend more time thinking about the pain—and this produces *fear*.

This fear can take many forms. It can be despair that they will never get better, or fear that the underlying condition is more serious than was first imagined. The effect of the fear, however, is merely to recreate and intensify the feelings of tension and anxiety. When this happens the mind focuses back on the pain with the result that the pain is reinforced.

This triad of anxiety, isolation and fear (Figure 4) may

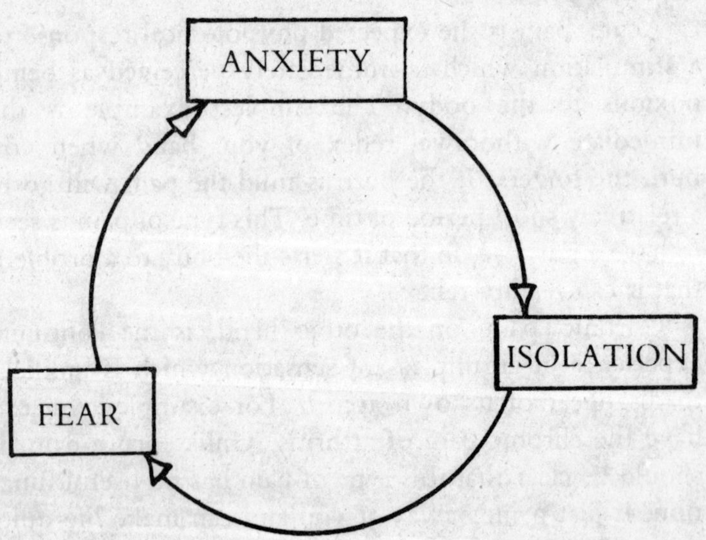

Figure 4. The Vicious Circle of Pain

well be the crux of many people's chronic pain. Indeed, it can explain why many chronic pain sufferers do not respond to pain-killers. The vicious circle becomes so strong that the symptomatic removal of the pain just doesn't work. In such cases it may be that breaking the circle between any of the above-mentioned links may be the approach which will work.

Homoeopathy and pain

There are no such things as homoeopathic pain-killers, just as there are no homoeopathic antibiotics, tranquillisers or stimulants. In homoeopathy we try to match the remedy profile to the patient profile. If pain is part of that profile then the corresponding remedy may help for that individual.

From the above discussion it should also be clear that the triad of anxiety, isolation and fear are worth tackling in any situation of chronic pain. By focusing upon the outlook, or the negative mental states ONE CAN USE THE BACH FLOWER REMEDIES TO BREAK THE LINKS IN THE VICIOUS CIRCLE OF PAIN.

As a first step I would suggest examining the feelings which the pain engenders then specifically look at the remedies under Dr Bach's headings for fear, loneliness and despondency and despair, as outlined in Chapter Six. There may of course be other associated negative states which crop up and these can also be combated.

Consider the type of pain

Orthodox medicine seems strangely unconcerned about the way the individual perceives his pain. Most research focuses upon ways of measuring pain, as if pain was some sort of thing which had a definite range and which could be calibrated. The fact that six patients suffering from exactly the same condition can describe their pain in six different ways seems to pass unnoticed.

In homoeopathy, on the other hand, we are acutely conscious of the type of pain that is being experienced. Indeed, the type of pain may well indicate the particular remedy, by virtue of the fact that many of the remedies have characteristic pain qualities.

Burning pains characterise the following remedies:

Aconite
Apis
Arnica
Arsenicum album
Belladonna
Bryonia
Causticum
Euphrasia
Graphites
Mercurius
Natrum muriaticum
Nitricum acidum
Nux vomica
Phosphorus
Pulsatilla
Rhus tox
Spigelia
Sulphur

Boring pains

Argentum nitricum
Belladonna
Pulsatilla
Spigelia

Bursting pains

Belladonna
Bryonia
Calcarea carbonica
Causticum
Ignatia

Nux vomica
Nitricum acidum
Sepia

Cutting pains

Belladonna
Calcarea carbonica
Colocynth
Drosera
Lycopodium
Nux vomica
Natrum muriaticum
Pulsatilla
Sulphur
Zincum metallicum

Cramp pains

Belladonna
Calcarea carbonica
Colocynth
Cuprum metallicum
Magnesia phos
Natrum muriaticum
Phosphorus
Phosphoric acidum
Sulphur
Zincum metallicum

Splinter-like pains

Argentum nitricum
Hepar sulph
Nitricum acidum

Sore pains

Arnica
Belladonna
China
Drosera

Hepar sulph
Nux vomica
Natrum muriaticum
Phosphorus
Rhus tox
Sulphur
Zincum metallicum

Throbbing pains
Aconite
Calcarea carbonica
Nitricum acidum
Phosphorus
Pulsatilla
Sepia

Consider what makes it better or worse

The modalities, the factors which aggravate or improve symptoms are very important when dealing with pain.

Worse for thinking about
Baryta carb
Causticum
Gelsemium
Nux vomica

Better for movement
Dulcamara
Lycopodium
Phosphoricum acidum
Rhododendron
Rhus tox
Ruta

Worse for movement
Aconite
Apis
Arsenicum album
Belladonna
Bryonia
Gelsemium
Hypericum
Lachesis
Magnesia phosphorica
Natrum muriaticum
Nux vomica
Phosphorus
Spigelia
Sulphur
Zincum metallicum

Better for lying down
Bryonia
Nitricum acidum
Nux vomica

Worse for lying down
Arsenicum album
Belladonna
Drosera
Lycopodium
Pulsatilla
Rhus tox
Zincum metallicum

Better for rubbing
Calcarea carbonica
Natrum muriaticum
Phosphorus
Pulsatilla
Rhus tox
Thuja
Zincum metallicum

Worse for the cold
Arsenicum album
Baryta carb
Causticum
China
Dulcamara
Graphites
Hypericum
Lycopodium
Magnesia phosphorica
Nitricum acidum
Phosphorus
Ranunculus
Rhus tox
Sepia
Spigelia

Better for the cold
Bryonia
Gelsemium
Pulsatilla

Better for the damp
Aconite
Belladonna
Bryonia
Causticum
Hepar sulph
Nitricum acidum
Nux vomica
Zincum metalicum

Worse for the damp
Bryonia
Dulcamara
Gelsemium
Hypericum
Thuja

Worse for a change in the weather
Dulcamara
Phosphorus
Ranunculus
Rhododendron
Rhus tox

Worse for wet weather
Arsenicum album
Calcarea carbonica
Dulcamara
Pulsatilla
Rhododendron
Rhus tox

Summary

Pain is a complex problem which has to be looked at on several levels. Always think about the outlook on life to assess negative mental states, aiming in particular at breaking the vicious circle of pain by use of the Bach Flower Remedies. Then examine the type of pain and consider whether it has any obvious modalities. If it does and you find a listed homoeopathic remedy then check its characteristics in the section on Materia Medica.

10

Arthritis and Rheumatism

What passes under the name 'rheumatism' is in fact a pretty mixed bag of conditions. It includes various diseases which affect joints, bones and soft tissues. Some are more debilitating and more serious than others, so they should be diagnosed by a professional.

At this point we will look at several of these conditions to get some idea of the range.

Joint disorders

Rheumatoid Arthritis This is a connective tissue disorder which can affect all parts of the body, but predominantly the synovial membranes of joints. When it is present in the Third Age it has usually been with the individual for many years. It mainly affects the hands, feet, knees and elbows, often causing quite marked deformity and instability in the joints.

Osteoarthritis This is more common in the Third Age. It is the arthritis of wear and tear. All joints can be affected, most usually the spine, hips, knees and hands. By the age of 65 years 80–90 per cent of the population have X-ray changes of osteoarthritis, but only 20 per cent suffer pain from it.

Gout Is caused by the accumulation of uric acid crystals in joints, classically the big toe, but also in the knee. Diuretic tablets can provoke an attack.

Bone disorders

Osteomalacia This is a generalised bone disease which affects about 5 per cent of people in the Third Age. There is a lack of calcium in the bones caused by a lack of Vitamin D. It produces severe pain in the bones, muscle weakness and a characteristic 'waddle.' Sufferers may find climbing stairs and combing their hair difficult. The good news is that it is a correctable condition after diagnosis.

Osteoporosis This bone disorder has been heralded as the modern epidemic. It is a generalised loss of bone mass which affects about 20 per cent of women in the Third Age. The critical time to lose this bone mass is around the menopause, although it can also be caused by steroids, poor calcium intake and immobilisation in bed for long periods. It produces fragility of bones, especially of the wrist and thigh bones.

Paget's Disease This is a bone disorder characterised by the laying down of new bone in a chaotic fashion. This results in gross thickening and deformity of the skeleton. It causes pain (in 5 per cent of people with the condition), deafness from squashing of the acoustic nerves, brittleness of affected thickened bones, sciatica, and possibly problems with mobility. It is another condition which needs proper diagnosis because of the effectiveness of orthodox treatment.

Malignant conditions of bone It also has to be said that several types of cancer can spread to bone—notably, leukaemia, lung, testicle, ovary, breast, thyroid and prostate. If bones are involved, and they can be the first presentation of the underlying disease, then extreme pain is caused.

FOR THIS REASON ANY SUDDEN SEVERE PAIN IN THE BACK, SPINE OR LIMBS SHOULD BE TREATED SERIOUSLY AND A MEDICAL OPINION SOUGHT.

Soft tissue disorders

Polymyalgia rheumatica This is a condition which causes inflammation in the muscles of the shoulder and pelvic girdles. They become extremely painful, exquisitely tender and unresponsive to ordinary pain-killers. Again a medical opinion should be sought, because it can often progress into the condition of *Temporal Arteritis* (not to be confused with 'arthritis'). This is quite dangerous, because it affects the blood vessels in the scalp and eyes, at its worst producing sudden blindness. It is characterised by a thumping headache.
FOR THIS REASON ANY SUDDEN THUMPING HEADACHE, ATTENDED BY MUSCULAR PAIN AND TENDERNESS MUST BE REGARDED AS SERIOUS AND A MEDICAL OPINION SOUGHT URGENTLY.

Homoeopathic remedies

Such is the importance of many of these conditions that I feel it necessary for the individual to have a professional diagnosis first. Once done, homoeopathic remedies can go a long way to alleviating pain and stiffness.

FACIAL PAIN

Facial pain can be almost unbearable. It can be caused by a whole host of conditions ranging from sinusitis, through arthritis in the tempero-mandibular joint (the jaw joint) to Trigeminal neuralgia. The most common remedies which I use are as follows:

Aconite—especially when caused by cold winds or draughts.

Arsenicum album—when the pain tends to be episodic, at regular intervals and burning.

Colocynth—when the pain is cutting, cramping or tearing. May be worse if angry, or have started when had some powerful negative emotion. Usually affects left side.

Magnesia phos—when the pain is cramping or twitching. Tend to be quite placid by nature. Usually affects right side.

Ranunculus bulbosus—when the pain is burning and itching, mainly above the eyebrow. Especially if the pain has followed an attack of shingles.

Spigelia—when the pains are boring or bursting. Tends to affect left temple. May also get palpitations.

NECKACHE

Aconite—for sudden stiffness after being in a draught.

Magnesia phos—for sudden cramping pain with a twitching sensation.

Rhus tox—for pain and stiffness which is better for movement.

BACKACHE AND ARTHRITIS

Arnica—when there is a bruised feeling in joints, or after injury to an arthritic joint.

Argentum nitricum—for anxious, clumsy types who fall then get a flare-up of their arthritis.

Baryta carbonica—when there is burning pain in joints. Worse for the cold, for washing and for thinking about.

Bryonia—for flare-ups where keeping still makes the pain bearable. Any movement aggravates it.

Causticum—if contractures have started to develop.

Dulcamara—for flare-ups after a change in the weather, particularly if it turns cold and damp.

Pulsatilla—if the pains tend to flit from joint to joint.

Rhododendron—worse when storms approach. It is like a barometer. Tend to be fearful of thunderstorms.

Rhus tox—for pain and stiffness, better for movement.

Ruta—if ganglia and nodules are present. May feel that you have overdone it and strained the part.

SCIATICA

This is a type of nerve root pain which passes down the buttock and leg to the foot. Again, it is a pain which needs to be diagnosed by a professional.

Arsenicum album—for burning pain down the leg. May have cramping in the calves.

Colocynth—cutting, cramping or tearing pains running down the legs. More usually on the left side. May be worse if angry.

Lycopodium—when it is worse lying on the affected side. Usually affects the right.

Magnesia phos—for cramping, twitching or 'electric shock' type pains shooting down the leg. Usually placid types. Usually affects the right side. Feet may feel tender.

Rhus tox—when it is worse for cold and damp. Better for moving around.

BURNING FEET

Graphites—for burning sensation in the soles. Worse for movement.

Phosphorus—for burning sensation in the soles. Worse for a change in the weather. Worse for the cold. Better for rubbing.

Pulsatilla—for feet and legs feeling heavy. Feet may actually seem to be inflamed. Worse when the feet hang down (out of bed).

Sulphur—when there is a burning sensation of the feet, which improves by them being dangled out of bed at night.

GOUT

Lycopodium—when one foot feels cold and the other is hot. This does not only apply at the time of the acute flare-up of gout.

Pulsatilla—when the pains have flitted from joint to joint.

11

Disorders of the Heart and Lungs

Problems of both the heart and lungs are common in the Third Age. A quarter of people in the Third Age have ischaemic heart disease, either symptomless or producing angina, abnormal heart rhythms or heart failure. In addition, chronic bronchitis, emphysema, acute chest infections and cancer of the lung all increase in frequency the older one grows.

SINCE THESE ARE ALL SERIOUS CONDITIONS A MEDICAL DIAGNOSIS SHOULD BE ESTABLISHED FOR ALL CASES.

Homoeopathic treatment should not take the place of conventional treatment, but can be used in conjunction with orthodox medication, with your doctor's knowledge.

UNDER NO CIRCUMSTANCES SHOULD YOU DISCONTINUE ORTHODOX MEDICATION UNLESS ADVISED TO DO SO BY YOUR DOCTOR.

SEE NOTES ABOUT POTENCY AND DOSAGE AT THE BEGINNING OF PART 3.

Disorders of the heart

The heart is the pump which circulates blood around the body. It itself is unable to extract oxygen out of the blood which passes through it, so it has to be supplied by special arteries which carry oxygen to its muscle tissue. Ischaemic heart disease is the name given to the problem of the heart not getting enough oxygen, when the coronary arteries become narrowed and impede the flow of oxygenated blood to its tissues.

A myocardial infarction, coronary thrombosis or 'heart attack' occurs when there is a sudden blockage of one of the coronary arteries, resulting in sudden severe pain (in the Third Age they can be surprisingly painless) and permanent scarring of the part of the heart supplied by that coronary artery. They can, of course, be fatal so it makes sense to try to prevent them by not smoking, not overeating and taking appropriate exercise. (See Chapter Five.)

ANGINA

Angina pectoris is caused by cramp in the heart muscle when it does not get enough oxygen. The pain is typically in the central chest with radiation down the left arm. Medical advice should always be followed, but people who regularly suffer from it might benefit from the following supplementary homoeopathic remedies. Of course, if an anginal attack is prolonged or does not respond to the usual tablets or nitrate spray then medical aid should be sought urgently.

Aconite—if attacks are brought on by draughts. If there is accompanying fear and panic.

Arsenicum album—if attacks come on at periodic episodes. The pain seems to burn and may radiate up the back of the neck to the occiput. The attacks are always accompanied by anxiety.

Cactus—if the attacks are always vice-like.

Lachesis—if the attacks produce the desire to loosen clothing, particularly around the neck. There is a bloated sensation. Usually talkative types of people.

Spongia—if there is accompanying perspiration, fear of death and the sensation that the heart is swelling inside the chest.

PALPITATIONS

This is the sensation of an abnormal rhythm. This may be a racing sensation, an irregularity or a feeling of having missed a beat.

Arsenicum album—for palpitations which start on getting up in the morning. They are always associated with anxiety.

Baryta carb—for palpitations which are worse for lying on the left side. Thinking about them makes them come on.

Natrum muriaticum—for attacks that vary. Sometimes the pulse may be very slow, at other times it may race. Helps to lie down. Usually these people crave salt in their diet.

Rhus tox—for an irregular feeling, or sensation of dropping a beat. Worse while sitting, but eases if moves around.

Spigelia—for a sensation of racing heartbeat, worse for movement. Tends to come on in bed. Eased by lying on right side with head propped up.

HEART FAILURE

We tend to think of the heart as a double pump. The right side sends blood to the lungs and the left side receives it back from there before sending it out around the rest of the body. Both sides of the heart can 'fail' to function as a pump, the result being that fluid accumulates in different parts of the body.

When the left side fails—acute left ventricular failure—there is sudden onset of breathlessness due to fluid accumulating in the lungs. Often this will happen at night. THIS NEEDS EMERGENCY MEDICAL TREATMENT.

The right side of the heart tends to fail gradually—congestive cardiac failure—producing swelling of the liver and the accumulation of oedema, fluid in the feet and ankles. Again medical treatment is necessary, but homoeopathic remedies may help considerably.

Arsenicum album—when there is great anxiety. There is a feeling of great exhaustion, restlessness and burning over the swollen ankles.

Cactus—if there are frequent vice-like anginal attacks. There is swelling of the hands and ankles, even when the fluid is only starting to accumulate.

Lachesis—when there is a tight sensation all over. There is a desire to loosen clothes. There may be a slightly bloated, blue or purplish appearance. They feel hot and are worse after a sleep.

Disorders of the lungs

Chronic obstructive airways disease (COAD) is the name given to cover a group of conditions, all of which impair the efficiency of the lungs as organs responsible for the exchange of gases between the body and the external environment.

The differentiation between chronic bronchitis and emphysema is difficult on clinical grounds. Chronic bronchitis refers to persisting inflammation of the air passageways in the lungs together with a persistent productive cough, which has been present for at least three months. Emphysema refers to loss of functioning lung tissue through previous damage. Both of these conditions represent the 'irreversible' end of COAD, in that bronchodilator drugs cannot open up the airways to improve efficiency and relieve breathlessness.

Asthma is the 'reversible' end of COAD, in that bronchodilator drugs can improve the breathing.

It is important to have these adequately diagnosed. In particular, with any history of breathlessness and persisting cough in the Third Age it is important to rule out any malignancy.

SINCE THESE ARE ALL SERIOUS CONDITIONS A MEDICAL DIAGNOSIS SHOULD BE ESTABLISHED FOR ALL CASES.

As with disorders of the heart homoeopathic treatment should not take the place of conventional treatment, but can be used in conjunction with orthodox medication, with your doctor's knowledge.

COUGH

Since a cough is the most common lung symptom in the Third Age we shall look at the different types and the remedies which are indicated.

DRY NON-PRODUCTIVE COUGHS

Aconite—for hard, dry coughs brought on by the cold.

Baryta carbonica—for dry, suffocative coughs. Worse every time the weather changes.

Belladonna—for dry, tickling coughs which come in spasms. Worse at night. The larynx usually feels sore.

Bryonia—for dry coughs associated with soreness in the chest. Worse for movement, eating or drinking.

Calcarea carbonica—for dry coughs with pain in the larynx. Worse at night.

Pulsatilla—for dry coughs worse in the evening and night. Worse for entering a warm, stuffy room. Better for sitting up. Better for the open air.

Spongia—for dry, barking coughs. Worse before midnight. Better for eating or drinking.

LOOSE PRODUCTIVE COUGHS

Ipecachuana—when the choking cough leads to retching of phlegm, followed by nausea and vomiting.

Mercurius—for coughs productive of yellow phlegm. Worse for the warmth of the bed. Worse at night. Worse for wet weather.

Sepia—for a dry cough (if any) during the day, but productive at night.

SPASMODIC COUGHS

Cuprum metallicum—for spasms of coughing with a constricting feeling in the chest. Better for drinking cold water.

Magnesia phos—for spasmodic coughs which are worse for lying down.

12

Abdominal Ailments

As the digestive tract ages it becomes more susceptible to diseases of all sorts. Some of these can be serious, so an early medical opinion and diagnosis is important in the following situations:

- **Sudden severe abdominal pain.**
- **Vomiting, especially if accompanied by abdominal distension.**
- **Weight loss which is not from deliberate dieting.**
- **Alteration in the normal bowel habit, either with diarrhoea or constipation.**

Where a recurrent condition has been diagnosed medically, homoeopathic remedies can be used to supplement orthodox treatment.

DIFFICULTY SWALLOWING (Dysphagia)

This symptom must always be diagnosed by a professional, because of the danger of missing a serious condition.

China officinalis—for when the throat feels tender. Food tastes too salty.

Gelsemium—when there is difficulty swallowing warm food. Itching in the palate and a constant sensation of having a lump in the throat.

Ignatia—if the difficulty starts following a bereavement or emotional trauma. Swallowing liquids may be harder than solids.

Lachesis—when there is a bloated sensation in the throat and a bluish tinge to the complexion.

Nitricum acidum—when there is a splinter sensation in the throat.

HEARTBURN

This symptom refers to the burning sensation as stomach acid is squirted into the oesophagus from the stomach. It is therefore felt rising through the chest up to the back of the throat.

Many people take antacids, either bought over the counter or prescribed by their doctor. While one should not stop orthodox medication except in consultation with your doctor, it should be noted that antacids will prevent homoeopathic remedies from working if they are taken within half an hour of each other.

Calcarea carbonica—for cramps in the stomach, loud belching and burning heartburn. May get sour taste in mouth after belching. Milk disagrees (whereas it usually helps heartburn).

Lycopodium—for burning heartburn with regurgitation after only small meals. The burning only reaches to the Adam's Apple, but goes on burning for hours despite antacids, milk or water.

Pulsatilla—for heartburn when the taste of the food remains for a long time afterwards.

INDIGESTION (Stomach upset)

This is a symptom which for the purpose of this book is defined as arising from the stomach. It therefore tends to produce sensations felt in the upper abdomen.

Argentum nitricum—for nausea, gnawing discomfort in the upper abdomen and retching of mucus. Craving for sweet things.

Nux vomica—when the stomach is easily upset by rich

foods, alcohol and noisy environments. Classically comes on about two hours after food.

Pulsatilla—when there is nausea and great tightness of the upper abdomen after a meal. May feel like a stone in the stomach. Nearly always thirstless.

Sulphur—Burning pain in the upper abdomen. Usually comes on about an hour after food. Tends to feel faint with a sinking feeling in the stomach at about 11 a.m.

COLIC

This symptom is a specific type of pain resulting from spasm in a hollow organ, usually the small or large bowel. Unlike 'indigestion' (as used in this book) it is more likely to be felt in the middle or lower abdomen.

If it is sudden and severe then a medical opinion should be sought, lest it indicates the start of an urgent condition which might necessitate surgery. In such a situation homoeopathy has no part to play in the Third Age.

On the other hand, for recurrent known conditions homoeopathic remedies can be very beneficial.

Bryonia—for colic which is better for lying still. Worse for the heat of a hot water bottle.

Colocynth—for cramping, cutting pains which start after anger or deep emotions. Very restless.

Magnesia phos—for colic which is better for the heat of a hot water bottle.

CONSTIPATION

This refers to infrequent, difficult and sometimes painful evacuation of the bowels. Often the motions are very hard.

This is extremely common in the Third Age. It may be due to:-

ageing changes in the bowel
poor diet with low fibre intake

unsatisfactory toilet arrangements
immobility
disease of the bowel
side effects of drugs—e.g., Aluminium compounds, calcium salts, pain-killers.

ANY ALTERATION IN BOWEL HABIT COULD BE VERY SERIOUS, SO A MEDICAL OPINION SHOULD BE SOUGHT SWIFTLY.

Diet One should try to eat plenty of fibre. This is found in wholegrain cereals, oats, fruit and vegetables. Wholemeal bread is preferable to white bread, and digestive biscuits are preferable to other types.

Fluids People often restrict their fluid intake because of a fear that they may retain it, thereby causing swollen ankles, frequent bladder voiding, etc. In fact one should ensure an adequate fluid intake otherwise the body will conserve fluid, by removing it from the intestinal contents as they pass through the large bowel. This is one of the potential causes of constipation.

Immobility Prolonged bed rest has dire effects upon the bowel.

Poor mobility may tend to make individuals ignore their 'call to open their bowels.' By doing this one can set up the vicious circle which tends to create constipation.

Toilet arrangements should be adequate. If necessary your doctor can assess whether any aids would help.

Drugs In most research studies on people in the Third Age up to 50 per cent have been found to be taking regular laxatives. Often these are taken to counteract the constipating effects of other drugs. Your family doctor can always advise about this.

YOU SHOULD NOT STOP ANY MEDICATION WITHOUT MEDICAL ADVICE.

Homoeopathic treatment of constipation

Bach Flower Remedies

It is a fact that people in the Third Age often become preoccupied with their bowels. It is of course sensible to take measures to guard against constipation, but if one actually becomes obsessed then one's whole well-being can be affected. If a negative mental state arises then it is worth considering remedies like:

Mimulus—if fearful of developing a disease such as cancer.

White Chestnut—if unable to think of anything else. Totally obsessed.

Crab Apple—if feelings of self-disgust appear.

Alumina—for constipation, producing hard, knotty motions which may provoke bleeding.

Baryta carbonica—for constipation with hard, knotty motions.

Bryonia—when the motions are large, hard and seem to burn as they are passed. Constipation tends to be worse if there has been a lot of travelling. Drinking large amounts seems to have no effect.

Calcarea carbonica—usually the individual feels better if they are constipated.

Nitricum acidum—when it is painful to open the bowels. There is a feeling that one is passing sharp sticks.

Silica—the motion seems to stick in the rectum. Great straining produces a stinging sensation. When the motion is partially expelled, it often recedes inside again.

HAEMORRHOIDS (Piles)

It is important to have haemorrhoids confirmed by a doctor before beginning any sort of treatment. This is especially the case if bleeding occurs from the rectum, since cancer of the rectum must be excluded.

Aloe—if there are haemorrhoids present like 'grapes.' They tend to be very sore and there is a constant uncertainty as to whether gas or motions will be passed.

Baryta carbonica—if the haemorrhoids prolapse when urine is being passed.

Causticum—when the back passage is sore, burning and itching.

Hamamelis—if the back passage feels bruised. This remedy can be used in either oral form or applied as an ointment.

Hypericum—when the back passage is extremely sensitive and tender. They may bleed easily on touching them.

Nitricum acidum—when there is a splinter-like sensation.

Thuja—when there are warts present. (But have them confirmed; do not assume that they are warts.)

13

Urinary Problems

Problems with the urinary system are extremely common. Not only does the muscular tone in the urinary organs decrease, but the efficiency of the kidneys drops off with increasing age. By the age of 85 years the blood flow to the kidneys is only half that of a young adult's. Similarly, the functioning kidney tissue is reduced by half. These two effects mean that a great strain can be imposed upon the remaining functional tissue as the kidneys strive to maintain the integrity of the body's internal fluid balance.

In addition, prostatic enlargement in men and a tendency for the vaginal wall to weaken in women can create problems in the way the bladder functions.

Danger symptoms

As with problems of the abdomen it is important to seek a swift medical diagnosis if any of these symptoms occur:

Unexpected weight loss
Passage of blood in the urine
Incontinence
Retention of urine (Emergency)
Sudden severe pain in the loins or lower abdomen (Emergency)

Infections of the urinary system are common. Some studies have shown that the rate of infection in elderly people living at home can be as high as 20 per cent, the majority of whom are quite unaware of it. The potential danger, however, is that the infection could ascend from the bladder to the kidney to produce a 'pyelitis,' which could be catastrophic.

SUDDEN CHANGES IN THE WATERWORKS SHOULD BE ASSESSED BY A DOCTOR BEFORE STARTING ANY TREATMENT.

URINARY FREQUENCY

If the frequency is long-standing, and if investigations have excluded any serious cause then the following homoeopathic remedies can be helpful.

Baryta carbonica—constant desire to pass urine. May find that haemorrhoids come down when it is passed.

Causticum—when there is frequency both during the day and the night.

Nux vomica—when there is frequency, but little is passed. There is general irritability. Often itches during the process of passing water.

Sepia—where there is a bearing down sensation as the urine is passed.

BURNING WHEN PASSING URINE

Again, provided infections have been excluded:

Apis—where there is a burning and stinging sensation. The urine may seem very concentrated.

Argentum nitricum—where there is burning, itching and a splinter-like sensation. Urine is dark and scanty.

Arsenicum album—where the burning is so intense that it causes agitation. The sufferer cannot keep still.

Nitricum acidum—where the urine burns, stings and smells offensive (classically like horse's urine) in the absence of infection.

Sulphur—when there is burning on passing urine, but which lasts long after the urine has been passed.

INCONTINENCE

The involuntary passage of urine is a distressing symptom. In the Third Age it may well be that the problem is not true incontinence, but a difficulty in reaching the toilet in time. This needs to be considered.

Exercises are always worth doing to try to increase bladder tone in order to gain more control.

The first is simply to try to squeeze the anal sphincter closed. Just sit and try to squeeze your buttocks together. Then as you hold that position for five to ten seconds, try to force the anus tightly closed. Do not tire yourself doing it, but build up to doing it five times at each session. Aim at three sessions a day.

The second exercise is to be done every time you actually go to pass urine. Simply, don't pass all the urine at once. Try stopping in midstream for five seconds, then allow some more to come, then stop again for five seconds, then allow it all to flow. This will help to build up tone.

Apis—when there is burning, stinging and incontinence on coughing.

Causticum—when the urine is passed frequently both day and night, and when it may be passed unnoticed by the individual.

Natrum muriaticum—when passes small amounts when coughing, laughing or straining. Stress incontinence. Craves salt.

Sepia—if passes urine involuntarily during sleep.

PROSTATE TROUBLES

Enlargement of the prostate gland in men increases in frequency with age. Difficulty in passing urine must always be investigated.

CANCER OF THE PROSTATE IS THE COMMONEST CANCER IN MEN IN THE THIRD AGE.

Indeed, because of this any man in his 80s or 90s who has been previously fit, should have a medical check if they start to feel generally unwell.

Benign prostatic enlargement may need surgery, but homoeopathic remedies might help the symptoms.

Baryta carbonica—when there is burning on passing urine in the presence of enlargement of the prostate.

Calcarea carbonica—for large 'doughy' men. May pass urine with a white sediment.

Silica—when there is a discharge from the penis when straining to open the bowels.

Thuja—when there is a frequent and urgent need to pass urine. The individual may be prone to warts and like drinking tea.

14

Women and Menopause

The menopause can be a traumatic time for many women. It marks the cessation of the reproductive part of their lives, so it is a time of great change. There are alterations in the hormone levels as the ovaries stop producing eggs, there is a loss of bone substance (which may produce osteoporosis) and there is a psychological adjustment to be made.

The main culprit in this time of change seems to be the hormone 'oestrogen.' As it falls during the menopause it causes menopausal flushing, vaginal dryness and soreness. There is also a complicated relationship with the metabolism of calcium and other minerals which may result in bone loss and osteoporosis.

Hormone Replacement Therapy (HRT) is now widely advocated as women approach and pass through the menopause, in order to minimise problems like flushing and vaginal soreness, and to prevent osteoporosis. Not everyone can tolerate this treatment, and indeed not everyone chooses to have it.

There are things that individual women can do to minimise problems in both their menopause and their post-menopausal years.

STOP SMOKING

It really is never too late to stop. Although the mechanism has not been fully delineated, there is no doubt that cigarette smoking is a major risk factor for heart disease, all cancers and osteoporosis.

EXERCISE

Moderate exercise seems to be more beneficial than strenuous exercise (see Chapter Five). For a fit 70-year old a round of golf a week, a swim or a brisk walk would all be adequate. For a fit 80-year old a walk twice a week would be fine. For those who are less able and require walking aids (e.g. walking sticks, tripods or Zimmer frames) they should still strive to use them as much as possible, since a lot of energy is needed in order to travel less distance.

Listen to your body and do not attempt any exercise beyond your limits. Remember the decades. What is reasonable for an average 50-year old would be quite strenuous for an average 60-year old and so on. If in doubt about your limits have a chat with your doctor.

DIET

There are two main factors to boost in your diet:

Calcium
Phyto-oestrogens (plant oestrogens)

Calcium A recent conference in Copenhagen advised that women at the menopause should take in 1,000–1,500 mg of calcium daily. Once through it into the Third Age an intake of 800–1,000 mg would be adequate.

To give you some idea of the calcium content of foods, a pint of semi-skimmed milk contains about 650 mg; a 5 oz pot of yoghurt contains 240 mg; and 1 oz of Cheddar cheese contains about 200 mg.

It is important, however, not to exceed 1,500 mg daily in the Third Age (unless of course advised to by your doctor) because of the potential risk of developing kidney stones.

Phyto-oestrogens It has been known since the 1970s that some crops used for animal pasture have oestrogenic activity. It is also known that some plants contain natural chemicals—'phyto-oestrogens.'

In 1990 an Australian team looked at the effect of these naturally-occurring plant oestrogens on women who had passed through the menopause. In order to do this the women had their diets supplemented with soya flour, various sprouts and a small amount of linseed oil. They found a very beneficial effect upon the cells of the vagina, compatible with improved oestrogen activity.

In this context 'sprouts' are various pulses and seeds which are moistened and allowed to sprout, e.g. soya beans and red clover.

In addition to the phyto-oestrogens, pulses are also good sources of protein, Vitamins B and C. They also have smaller amounts of iron, magnesium and calcium.

Adding soya to the diet instead of some of the red meat, plus some of the other sprouts, e.g. lentils, two or three times a week may result in symptomatic improvement.

IT IS IMPORTANT THAT PULSES SHOULD ALWAYS BE COOKED TO DESTROY THE PHYTIC ACID AND TOXIC LECITHINS IN THEM, OTHERWISE THEY CAN PRODUCE A SEVERE GASTRO-ENTERITIS.

BREAST PROBLEMS

A medical opinion should be sought swiftly with any of the following problems:

Lumps in the breast
Eczema or a rash forming around the nipple
A discharge from the nipple

Breast checks either by self examination or at your doctor's is advisable every six months. The technique can easily be learned.

Bryonia—if the breasts simply feel heavy, sore and are better for pressure.

Lachesis—if there is aching pain in the breasts in the mornings. There is usually an aversion to wearing high neck-lines.

FLUSHING

This may persist well into the Third Age. It is indicative of the oestrogen lack. It may improve with phyto-oestrogen containing foods.

Aurum metallicum—if there are frequent hot flushes. The temperament is usually melancholic.

Lachesis—if the flushings are accompanied by nausea, a bloated sensation and even retching. Dislike of tight clothing.

Sepia—if the flushes are accompanied by a dragging down sensation in the abdomen.

Sulphur—if there is much perspiration.

VAGINAL DISCHARGE

Any discharge or bleeding from the vagina after the menopause must be diagnosed by a doctor to exclude anything serious.

Recurrent vaginal infections may be a symptom of undiagnosed diabetes mellitis, so this is another reason for seeking a medical opinion.

VAGINAL DRYNESS

This again is usually a feature of oestrogen withdrawal. It too may improve with phyto-oestrogen containing foods.

Hamamelis—when there is tenderness, dryness and itchiness.

Lycopodium—when there is dryness, discomfort worse between 4 p.m. and 8 p.m. There may be subdued spirits and a constant worried frown.

Natrum muriaticum—where there is dryness, worse in the morning. Usually the individual craves salt.

Nitricum acidum—where there is dryness and prickling, like splinters.

Sulphur—where there is burning, dryness and pain.

15

Skin Troubles

The skin ages as one grows older. The epidermis, the outer layer of cells becomes thinner. Below this, the dermis decreases in bulk from the age of 60 onwards. Within its substance elastic fibres are lost and the collagen alters, making the skin stiffer. All of this, combined with loss of water from the dermal tissues results in the skin losing its mechanical integrity, resulting ultimately in the ageing appearance of the skin.

Not all of the changes that take place, however, are purely due to biological ageing. In many cases environmental damage from ultra-violet radiation produces further wrinkling, and alteration in pigmented areas of the skin with resultant pre-malignant or malignant change.

Another significant factor which can age the skin is the use of steroid-containing creams. Incredibly effective though they are, it is at a cost. Often rather than settling a skin problem they suppress it, causing the body to deal with the problem in some other way. It may be that it merely becomes encapsulated, adding another shell or onion-layer to the disease pattern of the individual.

Skin cancers

Potentially dangerous skin changes are:-

Alteration in shape and size of a wart
Alteration in size or shape of pigmented moles
Growth of hairs on pigmented moles
Spontaneous bleeding of pigmented moles

All of these changes may indicate that a malignant melanoma is starting to grow. This is a potentially life-threatening condition, so any of these changes should be treated with suspicion. A medical diagnosis should be sought.

Not all skin cancers occur in pigmented moles. Basal Cell Carcinomas, the commonest skin cancers can grow anywhere on the skin surface, the most common place being on the face. They have a slightly raised edge and are usually circular. Left to their own devices they slowly erode the surrounding tissues away, hence their old name of 'Rodent Ulcers.' Any suspicious spots on the face should therefore always be diagnosed by a doctor.

The skin is the mirror of the mind

There is much truth in this old axiom. Think of how people blush with embarrassment, go white with fear, purple with rage and perspire with anxiety.

In homoeopathy it is recognised that disorders of the skin are merely external markers of a more fundamental illness within the patient. This being the case, the constitutional remedies seem to work best. If it is not possible to select this, however, then one should try to get the local remedy with the best match to the patient-profile.

The Bach Flower Remedies are a good starting point with any skin problem. Simply examine the outlook upon life, assess any negative mental states and start taking the appropriate remedy. With many skin rashes this alone may be sufficient to begin internal healing.

Homoeopathic remedies can either be used by mouth or topically as creams or ointments. Arnica, Calendula and hypericum are all available as creams.

Arnica cream—for bruises.

Calendula cream—for cuts, lacerations, abrasions, fissures and bed sores.

Hypericum cream—similar range to Calendula. Also useful for crushed fingers, nips, splinters.

All of these creams are available in 30g tubes and are worth having in the medicine cabinet.

DRY AND CRACKING SKIN

Alumina—for chapped, dry hands, a tendency towards brittle nails and severe itch. The itch may be so bad that the need to scratch is so intense as to draw blood.

Arsenicum album—for dry, burning, scaling skin.

Calcarea carbonica—for unhealthy looking skin that ulcerates easily.

Graphites—for dry, cracked skin around the nose, mouth and ears.

Natrum muriaticum—for dry skin on the hands, especially around the nails with resultant hangnails. Also cracks around joints.

Nitricum acidum—for dry cracks which bleed and crust over. Produce a stinging sensation around the nose.

Petroleum—for rough, hard, dry skin that tends to crack and leave deep fissures. Found on the palms of the hands and over the heels. Worse for the cold.

Sulphur—for dry, red, scaly skin that cracks. Often found in skin folds on the abdomen, under the breasts and in joint flexures.

ITCH

This is a curious symptom which results from the stimulation of nerves which transmit the sensation of fine touch and pain. There does not seem to be a separate nerve pathway for itch itself, the perception of itching being due to a curious combination of fine touch and pain stimulation. It would seem, therefore, that when the balance is predominantly made up of fine touch, one perceives the sensation as a tickle. When the balance is predominantly pain, the feeling is of itching.

Alumina—for chapped, dry hands, a tendency towards brittle nails and severe itch. The itch may be so severe that the need to scratch is so bad as to draw blood.

Anacardium orientale—for intense itching and mental irritability, especially if there is a tendency towards forgetfulness. There may be swearing which is out of character.

Arsenicum album—for dry, scaling, burning and itching skin. May be very restless because of it. Very neat individuals.

Calcarea carbonica—for unhealthy looking skin. May get nettle-rash (urticaria). Generally better for scratching.

Graphites—for dry skin that is so itchy that scratching may cause bleeding. Especially around the nose, mouth and ears.

Pulsatilla—for nettle-rash after eating rich food. It tends to flit around the body. Worse in stuffy rooms.

Sulphur—for burning, itching and red scaling skin. Worse for heat, washing or scratching.

Urtica urens—classically for nettle-rash (urticaria). Skin is hot, blotchy. For prickly heat.

SHINGLES

This condition is due to the flare-up of the chickenpox virus in a skin nerve, where it has been dormant ever since the individual had chickenpox. This can even be eighty years in the past.

Shingles is characterised by a skin rash and by pain. The rash is usually red, with the appearance of little blisters which burst and scab over. Typically it is restricted to only one side of the body. The pain, felt over the same area as the skin rash, can range from mild discomfort to excruciating agony. With luck both the rash and the pain should resolve in two to three weeks. In a small proportion of people, however, the pain can persist for a long time after the disappearance of the rash. This is called 'post-herpetic neuralgia.'

IF SHINGLES BREAKS OUT ON THE FACE IT IS IMPORTANT TO SEEK A MEDICAL OPINION, BECAUSE THERE IS A DANGER OF THE EYE BEING AFFECTED.

Arsenicum album—for burning pain with the rash. May be better for heat. Tendency to be very restless.

Lachesis—for shingles with a purplish rash. Tends to be extremely sensitive. May be better for cold. Talkative types.

Ranunculus bulbosus—for shingles with burning and intense itching. Worse for contact. Worse for movement.

Rhus tox—when there is great restlessness, better for movement. The pain is burning and accompanied by itching.

Thuja—for post-herpetic neuralgia.

WARTS

Calcarea carbonica—for warts on the face and hands which tend to itch.

Causticum—for warts around the nose and eyes. There is a tendency for them to bleed.

Natrum muriaticum—for warts on the palms.

Nitricum acidum—for large, craggy warts which feel itchy and prickly. There is a tendency for them to bleed when touched or washed.

Thuja—a good treatment for all types of wart. Often there is a great desire for tea.

ULCERS AND SORES

Arsenicum album—for skin ulcers or sores which burn. They often have an offensive discharge. There is general restlessness as a result.

Belladonna—when the ulcer or sore develops rapidly and is surrounded by redness. The pupils of the eyes may be dilated.

Lachesis—for ulcers or sores with a purplish appearance. They may make the individual angry.

Nitricum acidum—for skin ulcers or sores which bleed on touching and washing. They may prickle.

Silica—for skin ulcers or sores which are difficult to heal.

16

Faints, Falls and Shocks

Faints, falls, shocks and traumas are all quite common in the Third Age. It is well worth having a few well-selected homoeopathic remedies in the First Aid cupboard.

FOR MENTAL SHOCKS

This could be after hearing bad news, witnessing a trauma, suffering an injury or illness oneself.

Rescue Remedy—the composite Bach Flower Remedy for helping with the emotional state that accompanies any shock, panic, stress or panic. I always carry a bottle in my medical bag and would recommend everyone to have one in their cupboard.

Star of Bethlehem—for the shock of sudden news, bereavement or accidents.

Aconite—for physical or mental shock where the individual becomes agitated, excited, frightened or feverish. May develop a throbbing headache or palpitations.

FOR PHYSICAL SHOCKS

Aconite—for physical or mental shock where the individual becomes agitated, excited, frightened or feverish. May develop a throbbing headache or palpitations.

Arnica—for soft tissue injuries, such as bruises, sprains and strains. It will also remove the shock created by the injury. Indeed, a shock from an accident several years in the past can still exert an effect on the individual. In such cases Arnica will remove the shock and any chronic troubles arising from it.

It is also useful for more severe injuries and reduces the time of recovery after operations and broken bones.

Carbo vegetabilis—for collapses and faints. These should of course be dealt with by a professional, but a dose of Carbo veg while awaiting aid can often produce startling results.

Hypericum—for crushed fingers and toes, and any problem where there has been nerve damage.

BOTH THE 6c AND 30c POTENCIES CAN BE USED IN THE FIRST AID SITUATION. THEY CAN BE TAKEN EVERY FIFTEEN MINUTES UNTIL IMPROVEMENT BEGINS, THEN EVERY 2–4 HOURS FOR 24 HOURS.

TOPICAL TREATMENT

In addition to oral treatment the use of creams can be very useful in the first aid situation.

Arnica—for all bruises, strains and sprains where the skin has not been broken.

Calendula—for all cuts, grazes, fissures, bed sores and ulcers. Very small superficial burns may also benefit. It should be noted, however, that the more serious a burn the less pain may be noted. If in doubt seek medical aid.

Hypericum—crushed parts, penetrating injuries with thorns, splinters and bites.

Rescue Remedy Cream—the Bach Flower Remedy composite in cream form for external use. Useful for ulcers, cuts, burns (as with Calendula) and sprains.

PART THREE

Selecting Appropriate Remedies

The Correct Approach

It is important to remember the following points when taking homoeopathic remedies in tablet form.

- The tablets should not be handled, but should be flicked into the mouth from the lid of the container, or placed there with a spoon. This is because the effectiveness of the tablet is only on the surface, not mixed all the way through as is a conventional tablet.

- Two tablets should be taken at a time—but they must be sucked not swallowed.

- The tablets should not be taken within half an hour of tea, food, coffee, smoking or having brushed the teeth.

- The remedies will last for a long time, providing they are kept away from potent-smelling substances. They are best kept in a drawer, away from perfumes, spices, pot-pourri or moth-balls.

Two potencies are recommended—6c for local remedies and 30c for constitutional remedies. Both potencies are usually available from chemists who stock homoeopathic remedies, health food shops, or directly from homoeopathic suppliers (See useful addresses at the back of the book).

If the constitutional remedy is obvious from a study of the Materia Medica then this can be taken in 30c potency, two tablets three times a day at the start of any acute illness. *It should only be taken for three days.* If improvement starts within that time then the remedy should be stopped then and there. There is no point whatsoever in '*taking extra just to make sure.*' It should not be repeated unless the symptoms reappear.

The constitutional remedy can also be taken for three days at a time every three months as a booster.

If a high potency remedy is taken continuously for too long (more than three days) then there is a strong likelihood of producing an aggravation of symptoms.

Local remedies are useful if taken to deal with a specific problem. They are best taken in 6c, low potency. They can be repeated more frequently than high potencies, but again, they should be stopped once symptomatic improvement occurs. They should not be repeated unless the symptoms start to come back.

Matria Medica

This covers the remedy profiles of all the remedies included in this book.

As you will see, I have considered each remedy under the headings of mentals, modalities, likes and dislikes, disease tendencies and physical features, as discussed in Chapter 4. Characteristic features of the remedies will be emphasised in capital letters, e.g. the THIRST of Aconite.

The major 'Constitutional' remedies will be marked with an asterisk.

Although there are many, many more which are of value in the Third Age, I have restricted the number to avoid making the book too complicated, yet tried to ensure that the most useful ones (in my experience) are included.

Materia Medica

Remedy	Abbreviation
Aconite	Acon
Ambra grisea	Amb gris
Aloe	Aloe
Alumina	Alum
Anacardium orientale	Anac
Apis mellifica	Apis
Argentum nitricum	Arg nit
Arnica	Arn
Arsenicum album	Ars alb
Aurum metallicum	Aur
Baryta carbonica	Bar carb
Belladonna	Bell
Bryonia	Bry
Cactus	Cact
Calcarea carbonica	Calc carb
Causticum	Caust
China	Chin
Cocculus	Cocc
Coffea	Coff
Colocynthis	Coloc
Cuprum metallicum	Cup met
Drosera	Dros
Dulcamara	Dulc
Euphrasia	Euph
Ferrum metallicum	Ferr
Gelsemium	Gels
Graphites	Graph
Hamamelis	Hamam
Hepar sulph	Hep sulph
Hypericum	Hyper
Ignatia	Ign
Ipecacuanha	Ipecac
Kali phosphoricum	Kali phos

Lachesis	Lach
Lycopodium	Lyc
Magnesia phosphorica	Mag phos
Mercurius solubilis	Merc
Natrum muriaticum	Nat mur
Nitricum acidum	Nit ac
Nux vomica	Nux vom
Petroleum	Petrol
Phosphoricum acidum	Phos ac
Phosphorus	Phos
Pulsatilla	Puls
Ranunculus bulbosus	Ranun
Rhododendron	Rhod
Rhus toxicodendron	Rhus tox
Ruta graveolens	Rut
Sepia	Sep
Silica	Sil
Spigelia	Spig
Spongia	Spon
Staphisagria	Staph
Sulphur	Sulph
Thuja occidentalis	Thuj
Urtica urens	Urt
Zincum metallicum	Zinc

ACONITE
(Monkshood)

A good remedy for THE START OF ILLNESSES. Not very good for chronic illness.
Always RESTLESS.
THIRST becomes marked.
TINGLING, NUMBNESS of local parts and BURNING internal pains.

Mentals
Great fear and anxiety with any illness.

Forebodings of doom.
Fear of death.
Anxiety about the future.
Becomes restless.
Good imagination.
May feel clairvoyant.

Modalities
Better for open air.
Worse in warm rooms.
Worse in evenings and night.
Worse on getting out of bed.
Worse for dry, cold winds and draughts.
Worse for music.

Likes and dislikes
Thirst for cold water.

Disease tendencies
Eye inflammations.
Feverish illnesses brought on by shock, fright, draughts, and too much sun.

Physical features
Robust, good-coloured types.

ALOE

(Socotrine Aloes)

Useful if there has been a lot of medication given.
Very useful for weary people in the Third Age with ITCHING and BURNING discomfort in the back passage from HAEMORRHOIDS.
HAEMORRHOIDS like a bunch of grapes.
DIARRHOEA after eating or drinking.
Also may be useful in INCONTINENCE.

ALUMINA

(Aluminium oxide)

Alumina is a remedy against the toxic effects of aluminium. (See Chapter 8.)

There is general DRYNESS of mucous membranes.

There is WEAKNESS or even PARALYSIS of parts.

There is general SLUGGISHNESS of all functions.

Mentals

Depressed mood.

Fear that will lose the power of reason.

Variable mood.

Memory problems and poor concentration.

Always hurried, although time seems to drag.

Modalities

Worse in the mornings.

Worse for warm rooms.

Worse for eating potatoes.

Better for open air.

Better for damp weather.

Better one day, worse on the next.

Likes and dislikes

Unusual tastes for indigestible things.

Likes tea and coffee.

Likes fruit and vegetables.

Dislikes meat.

Dislikes potatoes.

Disease tendencies

Dry eyes.

Dryness of the membranes of the respiratory system, with cough, chronic catarrh and hoarseness.

Headaches over top of skull.

Constipation with hard knotty motions.

Dry, cracked, itching skin problems.
Itching of back passage.
Numbness, weakness and paralysis of limbs.

Physical features
Pale, dry and possibly cracked skin.
Thin builds.

AMBRA GRISEA
(Ambergis)

Useful for frail, trembling, tottering people in the Third Age.
EXTREMELY ANXIOUS.
FORGETFULNESS.
Weakness, coldness and NUMBNESS.
One-sided complaints.

Mentals
Dread of people.
Likes solitude.
Extremely shy.
Anxious in presence of others.
Concentration and memory poor early in the morning.
Seems to forget question they ask almost before the next is asked.
Depressed mood varying with flare-ups of temper.

Modalities
WORSE FOR MUSIC.
Worse in mornings.
Worse when routine is upset.
Better for movement.
Worse when in company or when being watched.

Disease tendencies
Vertigo (dizziness).

Memory problems.
Weakness of all systems with age.

Physical features
Weak, frail, thin types.

ANACARDIUM ORIENTALE
(Marking Nut)

Mentals Useful for MEMORY LOSS.
Unusual and unexpected SWEARING.
May have strong moral sense, so feel GUILTY.
May feel as if he is two people.
May feel possessed.
Easily offended.

Modalities
Better for lying on painful part.
Better for rubbing.
Better for eating.
Worse for heat.
Worse for washing or bathing with hot water.

Likes and dislikes
Likes milk and dairy products.

Disease tendencies
Sensations of a PLUG in the back passage, in the ear, in the nose.
May get dyspepsia of the stomach, better for eating.
May get intense ITCHING of the skin which makes the irritability worse.
DIMINUTION OF ALL SENSES.

Physical features
Pale face.
Blue rings around the eyes.

APIS MELLIFICA

(The Honey-Bee)

Useful when there is sudden SWELLING or PUFFINESS of tissues which comes on suddenly.
BURNING and STINGING and THROBBING pains.
Very TENDER and SENSITIVE to touch.
ABSENT THIRST

Mentals
Apathy and indifference.
Memory problems.
Jealousy.
Tearfulness.
Whining.
Hard to please.
Clumsiness.

Modalities
Worse for heat in any form.
Worse for touch and pressure.
Worse for sleep.
Better for uncovering and for cold water.

Likes and dislikes
Craving for milk.

Disease tendencies
Headaches, which stab and sting and are worse for movement.
Eye problems which sting and burn.
Spasmodic cough.
Itching skin. May have weals like nettle rash.
Acute flare-ups of arthritis which sting and burn.
Insect stings.
Urinary incontinence with stinging as the urine is passed.

***** ARGENTUM NITRICUM
(Silver nitrate)

ANXIETY and APPREHENSION.
SPLINTER-LIKE SENSATIONS.

Mentals
Anticipatory anxiety. Will worry for days before an engagement, appointment or event.
The anxiety causes DIARRHOEA.
Never feels that there is enough time. Always in a hurry.
Impulsive. May follow seemingly foolish impulses.
Fear of death.
Fear of heights with Lemming impulse, as if would like to jump off.

Modalities
Worse for heat.
Worse at night.
Worse for sweet things.
Worse for getting into any emotional state.
Better for belching.
Better for cold air.
Better for pressure.
Worse for concentration.

Likes and dislikes
Craves sweets and chocolate.
Likes salt.
Likes cheese.

Disease tendencies
Eyestrain.
Flatulence.
Diarrhoea.
Splinter-like sore throats and splinter-like pains.

Anxiety states.
HEADACHES with TREMBLING, worse for concentration.
TREMBLING and weakness of lower limbs.

Physical features
Thin builds.
May suit extroverted types who achieve because they fear failure so much.
May wonder why they put themselves in certain situations as they anticipate the event or whatever with fear, trepidation and diarrhoea.

ARNICA
(Leopard's Bane)

AFTER TRAUMA.
SORE, BRUISED FEELINGS.
SHOCK AFTER INJURY OR ACCIDENT.
A good first aid remedy, called 'Arnica the healer.'

Mentals
Indifferent.
Irritable.
Forgetful and absent-minded.
Fear of death.
GREAT FEAR OF BEING TOUCHED when have a pain.
Always says he feels well, even if very ill.

Modalities
Worse for touch.
Worse for motion.
Worse for damp.
Worse for alcohol.
BETTER FOR LYING DOWN

Likes and dislikes
Likes pickles.
Likes vinegar.
Dislike of meat.
Dislike of milk.

Disease tendencies
All traumas.
Will remove the shock created by an accident or injury, even if this happened years in the past. Chronic problems arising from that shock may clear up after treatment with Arnica.

Physical features
Maybe slightly melancholic.
Generally stoical types who minimise problems and dislike bothering their doctors.

***** ARSENICUM ALBUM
(Arsenic)

There is very marked FASTIDIOUSNESS.
There is PERIODICITY of symptoms (eg, symptoms tend to recur at regular intervals).
There are BURNING PAINS.
RESTLESSNESS is marked.
There is CHILLINESS.
Right-sided problems

Mentals
There is anxiety and anguish.
With illness there may be hopelessness, as if the feeling is that nothing can help.
The reaction is out of proportion to the condition and may become irritable.
May need to take to bed for the slightest of problems.
There is restlessness and agitation.

Soon exhausted.
NEAT in all things. Almost OBSESSIONAL. Appearance, clothes, house and garden—they all have to be tended and groomed.
FEAR OF THE DARK.
Thirsty.

Modalities
Worse for wet weather.
WORSE AROUND MIDNIGHT UNTIL 2 A.M.
Worse for cold, cold drinks or food.
Better for heat.
Better for warm drinks.

Likes and dislikes
Likes fat.
Likes small drinks.

Disease tendencies
Skin problems, psoriasis, dandruff, heart failure, watery head colds which cause sore red noses.

Physical features
Anxious, pale and thin.
Intelligent, quick-witted and perfectionist types.

AURUM METALLICUM
(Gold)

AILMENTS CAUSED BY GRIEF
There is CHILLINESS.
BORING PAINS.

Mentals
LACK OF CONFIDENCE.
DEPRESSION, possibly even suicidal.
Hate contradiction.

Can become hysterical and angry.
CRITICAL of everyone and everything.
Prefers own company and dislikes having to talk.
Noises cause anxiety.
Fear of men.
Often troubled with nightmares.

Modalities
Worse at night.
Worse for concentration.
Worse on waking.
Better for cold.
May get problems in Winter—'Seasonal Affective Disorder,' known as SAD.

Likes and dislikes
Craves alcohol.

Disease tendencies
Catarrhal problems.
Nose and ear problems.
Boring and tearing joint and bone pains.
Skin ulcers.

Physical features
May have a staring, melancholic appearance.

***** BARYTA CARBONICA
(Barium carbonate)

There is often ENLARGEMENT of GLANDS, cysts, lipomas (fatty lumps), nodules and the PROSTATE GLAND in men.
There is CHILLINESS.

Mentals
There is memory loss and difficulty in thinking.

Tendency to dwell on problems and past grievances.
Fear of things about to happen.
Confusion.

Modalities
WORSE FOR THINKING ABOUT PROBLEMS.
Worse for washing.
Worse lying on affected side.
Better in open air.

Likes and dislikes
Cold food.

Disease tendencies
Headaches which feel as if the brain is loose.
Recurrent sore throats with enlarged glands.
Lipomas and cysts.
Dry coughs.
Palpitations when lying on left.
Constipation with hard knobbly motions.
Haemorrhoids which come out when urine is passed.
Urinary frequency.
Prostate problems.

Physical features
Tendency to be overweight.
Dry wrinkled skin.

BELLADONNA
(Deadly Nightshade)

There is HOTNESS, REDNESS, THROBBING and BURNING.
It is an acute remedy.
There is no thirst.
The ailment comes on rapidly.
Right-sided problems.

ALL OF THESE FEATURES CAN BE THE RESULT OF A SEVERE BACTERIAL INFECTION AND NEED TO BE CHECKED OUT BY A PROFESSIONAL. THIS IS IMPORTANT BECAUSE SO MANY DANGEROUS INFECTIONS CAN START THIS WAY IN THE THIRD AGE.

Mentals
May seem delirious.
May be angry or furious.
All the senses seem to be acute.

Modalities
Worse for touch.
Worse for being jarred.
Worse for noise.
Worse for draughts.
Better sitting up.
Better for warm room.

Likes and dislikes
Dislike of meat.
Dislike of milk.
Worse for having a haircut.
Worse for getting head cold.

Disease tendencies
All sudden infections, as mentioned above. It can be used usefully as an adjunct to orthodox treatment.
Throbbing headaches.

Physical features
Strong types.
Vivacious when well, but knocked for six when ill and seem to go delirious.

BRYONIA
(Wild Hop)

DRYNESS runs through this remedy. There are dry mucous membranes, dry mouth, dry eyes, dry coughs and hard, dry motions.
Right-sided complaints.
STITCHING AND TEARING PAINS.
AILMENTS BROUGHT ON BY ANGER.
Excessive thirst.

Mentals
There is IRRITABILITY and anger.
Desires to be left alone when ill.
Poor memory.
Anxiety about death.

Modalities
WORSE FOR MOVEMENT of any kind.
WORSE FOR COLD WINDS.
Better for cold.
Better for being perfectly still.
All ailments better for pressure, except abdominal problems which are made worse.
Better for lying on painful side.
Better being perfectly still.
Ailments may start with first of the warm weather.

Disease tendencies
Headaches of a splitting or bursting nature. Better for pressure.
Arthritis and rheumatic pains which are better for being still.
Constipation.
Dry coughs and pleurisy.

Physical features
Dark skin and dark-haired (or previously so)

Good build, but not obese.

CACTUS
(Night-blooming Cereus)

Produces CONSTRICTING and VICE-LIKE pains. Ailments tend to be PERIODIC, or come at regular intervals.

Mentals
Melancholic.
Anxiety.
Pains are so bad that feels like screaming.

Modalities
Worse lying on left side.
Better in open air.
Better for pressure.

Disease tendencies
Headaches which are vice-like.
Angina pains which are vice-like.
Palpitations when walking.

***** CALCAREA CARBONICA
(Calcium carbonate)

There is CHILLINESS.
There is SLOWNESS.
There is CONGESTION of all types—of the heart, lungs, bowels.
There is SOFTNESS.

Mentals
Depression.
ALL SORTS OF FEARS—of the dark, impending doom, insanity and death.

Fear of strokes is common.
Anxiety worse in the evenings, producing palpitations.
Forgetfulness and confusion.
Forget what they have read soon after putting the book or magazine aside.
There is general slowness of thought.
There is a tendency to dwell on problems, often to the exasperation of friends, relatives and carers.
Talking about their problems makes them weep.
Dislike criticism or hard talking, which makes them anxious.

Modalities

WORSE FOR EXERTION—both physical and mental.
Worse for the cold in every form.
Worse for the damp.
Worse for standing.
Worse during the full moon.
Better for dryness and warm weather.
Better for lying on painful side.
Better for rubbing.
Better for lying on back.

Likes and dislikes

Dislikes meat.
Dislikes boiled food.
Dislikes fat.
Dislikes milk.
Likes indigestible things.
Likes eggs.
Likes salt.
Likes sweets.

Disease tendencies

Depression.
Chronic catarrh (Congestion).
Nasal polyps (Congestion).
Dry irritating cough (Congestion).

Constipation (Congestion)
Warts
Obesity
Backache.

Physical features

There is a flabby, doughy, soft appearance.

The handshake is floppy and the knuckles of the hands may appear as dimples, because of the soft, doughy appearance.

The feet tend to be cold and clammy.

There is a tendency to sweat on the head and chest.

*****

CAUSTICUM
(Potassium hydrate)

BURNING, BURSTING and TEARING PAINS.
PROGRESSIVE WEAKNESS leading to PARALYSIS.
In 'broken-down' constitutions in the Third Age.
Contractures.
Conditions caused by grief.

Mentals

Despair of recovery.
Fear of the dark.
Fear of doom.
Irritability.
Bereavement may cause illness.
Sympathetic to others.
Poor memory.
Concentration makes symptoms worse.

Modalities

WORSE FOR COLD WINDS.
Worse for motion.
Better in damp, warm weather.

Likes and dislikes

Upset by smell of food.
Worse for sweet foods.
Worse for coffee.

Disease tendencies

Paralytic problems, especially when single nerves are affected, e.g. Bell's palsy (Facial palsy).
Contractures of muscles and tendons.
Painful neck, brought on by the cold.
Tearing pains of muscles, joint and bones.
Stress incontinence, when coughing, sneezing, laughing and exertion cause urine to be passed involuntarily.
Haemorrhoids.
Warts, especially on the face and fingers.

Physical features

Broken-down appearance—sickly-looking, dark-eyed types who are 'rheumatic.'
Dark hair (or previously dark).

CHINA

(Cinchona bark)

A remedy for DEBILITY—from diarrhoea, blood loss, excess perspiration and excessive use of laxatives (i.e. from loss of body fluids).
PERIODICITY—complaints often come every other day.
There is CHILLINESS.

Mentals

Apathy.
Indifference.
Despair.
Can be deliberately hurtful to others when the mood takes them.

Thoughts whirl around the mind, causing insomnia.
Sudden, unexpected bursts of tears.

Modalities
WORSE FOR SLIGHTEST TOUCH.
Worse every other day.
Worse for losing fluids from the body.
Better for doubling up.
BETTER FOR FIRM PRESSURE.
Better for the open air.
Better for warmth.

Likes and dislikes
Dislikes milk.
Dislikes fruit.

Disease tendencies
BURSTING HEADACHES followed by TENDER SCALP, RELIEVED BY PRESSURE.
Abdominal distension not relieved by passing wind.
TINNITUS (ringing in ears)—sensitive to touch.
DEAFNESS associated with the tinnitus.

Physical features
Hollow eyed, blue rings around them and a yellow appearance to the sclera (BUT NOT JAUNDICE—it is not something which develops, but an appearance which has always been present).
Sweats around the nose.

COCCULUS
(Indian cockle)

DEBILITY FROM LACK OF SLEEP.
Good remedy for travel-sickness and VERTIGO
There is a sense of HOLLOWNESS of affected parts.

There is a sense of the affected parts having GONE TO SLEEP.

Mentals
CAPRICIOUS.
Gets very sad.
Bursts into song.
Slow on the uptake sometimes.
Fast speech.
Concerned for others.
SENSITIVE TO INSULTS OR CONTRADICTION.
Difficulty thinking and concentrating if has missed sleep.
Unable to find the right word.

Modalities
WORSE FOR EATING.
NAUSEA AT THE SMELL OF FOOD, especially when has vertigo.
WORSE FOR LACK OF SLEEP.
WORSE FOR MOTION.
Worse after emotional upset.

Likes and dislikes
Likes cold beer.
When nauseated, dislikes all food.

Disease tendencies
Painful contractures of the limbs, especially when affecting one side of the body.
Numbness of parts, as if they've gone to sleep.
Facial paralysis.
Confusion and poor memory.
Constant drowsiness with spasmodic yawning.

Physical features
Often some lameness, paralysis or weakness.
May be light-haired (or have been).

COFFEA
(Coffee)

There is HYPERSENSITIVITY to pain.
All pains seem intolerable.
There is abnormal activity of the brain. Mind-buzz.
Neuralgias.

Mentals

There is irritability.
The senses seem acute.
The mind buzzes with ideas.
Anxiety also comes swiftly and produces restlessness and anguish.
Insomnia because of the mind-buzz.

Modalities

WORSE FOR EXCESS EMOTIONS OF ALL SORTS (e.g. excitement, anger, joy)
Worse for strong smells.
Worse for open air.
Better for warmth.
Better for lying down.
Better for holding cold water in mouth.

Disease tendencies

HEADACHES LIKE A NAIL BEING DRIVEN INTO SKULL.
Insomnia.
Palpitations when excited, overjoyed or angry.
Anxiety and agitation.
Hypersensitive skin.

Physical features

Tall, lean types with a tendency to stoop.
Dark complexion.

COLOCYNTH

(Bitter cucumber)

Ailments which follow ANGER or INDIGNATION.
Often causes intense NEURALGIAS.
CRAMPING, CUTTING, CONSTRICTING and SPASM pains.
Agonising, DOUBLING-UP abdominal pains.
Symptoms often start on the LEFT SIDE.

Mentals
Restlessness.
Irritability.
Angry when questioned.
Indignation.
Quick to take offence.

Modalities
WORSE FOR ANGER.
Worse for indignation.
BETTER FOR DOUBLING-UP.
Better for hard pressure.

Likes and dislikes
Dislikes cheese.

Disease tendencies
Neuralgias—mainly LEFT-SIDED.
Sciatica—left sided.
Cramps relieved by lying on the affected side with the legs drawn up.

Physical features
Tendency to be overweight.
Offensive-smelling perspiration.
Contracted muscles.

CUPRUM METALLICUM
(Copper)

CRAMPING, CONSTRICTING and SPASM pains.
Symptoms often start on the LEFT SIDE.
Symptoms always feel EXTREMELY SEVERE.
COPPERY TASTE—'like old pennies.'

Mentals
Easily tired.
Has to keep on the go.
Confused when ill.
Gets fixed ideas in mind.
Often uses the wrong words.

Modalities
Worse in the evenings and at night.
Worse in the cold.
Worse for vomiting.
BETTER FOR COLD DRINKS.
Better for perspiration.

Likes and dislikes
Likes cold drinks.
Likes warm food.

Disease tendencies
All cramps—chest, abdomen, limbs or neuralgias.
Cramps often start in the fingers and toes.
Nausea, eased by drinking cold water.

Physical features
Bluish tinge to mouth and lips.
Complains of slimy, metallic, coppery taste.
Constant need to lick lips, so that the tongue darts in and out, reptilian fashion.

DROSERA
(Sundew)

SPASMODIC problems.
Hoarse voice.
ASTHMA WHEN TALKING.

Mentals
Nil in particular.

Modalities
WORSE AFTER MIDNIGHT.
Worse for laughing.
Worse for the warmth of the bed.
Worse for singing.
Worse for laughing.
Better for motion.
Better for sitting up.
Better for quiet.
Better for cold air.

Likes and dislikes
Dislikes citrus fruits.
Dislikes vinegar.

Disease tendencies
Laryngitis.
Coughs which are worse for lying down.
Asthma which is worse for lying down.
Family history of TB.

Physical features
Nil in particular.

DULCAMARA
(Bitter-sweet)

Ailments for CHANGE IN THE WEATHER.
Colds caused by cold, damp surroundings.

Mentals
Confusion—especially when there is a change in the weather.

Modalities
Worse at night.
Worse for the cold.
Worse for damp and rain.
Better for movement.
Better for heat.

Likes and dislikes
Likes cold drinks.
Dislikes all food when ill.

Disease tendencies
Itchy skin problems.
Warts.
Rheumatism—worse for weather changes.
Neuralgia—worse for weather changes.
Conjunctivitis.
Loss of voice.

Physical features
Nil in particular.

EUPHRASIA
(Eyebright)

STREAMING COLDS WITH BURNING SYMPTOMS.

Mentals
Nil in particular.

Modalities
Worse in evenings.
Worse indoors.
Worse for being in bed.
Worse for heat.
Worse for South winds.
Worse for light.
Better for dark.
Better for drinking coffee.

Likes and dislikes
Dislikes tobacco and smoking.

Disease tendencies
Catarrhal problems of the eyes and nose.
Watery eyes and nose.

Physical features
Tendency to have runny eyes with red rims.

FERRUM METALLICUM
(Iron)

There is CHILLINESS.
Tendency to develop a TEMPERATURE easily.
Tendency to flush or blush from emotion.
Tendency to BLEED EASILY.
Symptoms start while eating.

DEBILITY FROM LOSS OF FLUIDS.
THROBBING headaches.
Cold extremities.

Mentals
Extremely sensitive.
Low pain threshold.
SENSITIVE TO NOISE.
Restlessness.
Irritability.
Changeable moods.
Depression.
Anxiety.

Modalities
Worse sitting still.
Worse for cold.
Better for movement.
Better for heat.

Likes and dislikes
Dislikes fat.
Dislikes eggs.
Dislikes meat.
Dislikes sour fruit.
Voracious appetite or total lack of appetite.

Disease tendencies
Colds and respiratory infections.
Vertigo—especially if crossing water.
Throbbing headaches.
Diarrhoea and/or vomiting starting while eating.
Rheumatic pains—especially of the shoulders.
Varicose veins.
Nose bleeds—after emotions.

Physical features
Usually pale, anaemic-looking with 'flabby muscles.'

*****

GELSEMIUM
(Yellow jasmine)

The classic 'Flu' remedy.
There is great DROWSINESS with any ailment. There is nearly always the desire and need to lie down and sleep.
There is PROSTRATION, DIZZINESS and DULLNESS.
TIGHT, BURSTING HEADACHES.
Shivers up and down the spine.
Ailments from strong emotions—fear, anger, excitement.

Mentals
Wants to be left alone.
ANTICIPATORY ANXIETY—worries for days before an appointment, event, meeting.
Excitable nature.
Confusion and drowsiness.
Unable to control muscles when ill.

Modalities
Worse for damp weather.
Worse before storms.
Worse for strong emotions.
WORSE FOR THINKING ABOUT AILMENTS.
Worse in mornings.
Better for bending backwards.
Better for being still.
Better for passing a lot of urine.

Likes and dislikes
LACK OF THIRST.

Disease tendencies
Paralytic conditions.

Migraine, especially producing occipital headaches.
Vertigo.
Respiratory infections and classical 'flu,' when there is great prostration.
Diarrhoea in anticipation of some dreaded appointment, event or meeting.

Physical features
Heavy eyelids.
Flushed appearance.
Dusky skin.

*****

GRAPHITES
(Black lead)

Usually a female remedy.
Skin problems—tendency for wounds and cuts to FESTER.
CONSTIPATION with hard, knotty stools.
There is CHILLINESS.
ALTERNATING SKIN AND DIGESTIVE PROBLEMS.

Mentals
Timidity.
Indecisiveness.
Depression.
Tendency to fidget.
Anxiety.
MUSIC CAUSES WEEPINESS.
Often feels as if there are cobwebs on the face.

Modalities
Worse for heat.
Better in the dark.
Better for wrapping up.
Better for surrounding noise.
Better for eating.

Likes and dislikes
Dislikes meat.
Dislikes seafood and fish
Dislikes sweets.
Dislikes hot drinks.

Disease tendencies
Styes.
Skin problems—all injuries tend to fester and take a long time to heal. Get cracked, dry skin around the nostrils, lips and behind the ears. May also get discharges which are thick, like honey. Crusting may take place afterwards.
Nail problems.
Stomach problems and indigestion, relieved by eating.
Nose-bleeds.
Chilblains.

Physical features
Obesity.
Unhealthy skin.
Red-faced.
Eyelids often red and swollen.
Sore nose with cracked skin around it
Bad breath.

HAMAMELIS
(Witch hazel)

CONGESTED BLOOD VESSELS, VARICOSE VEINS AND HAEMORRHOIDS.
INJURIES.
Hammering headaches.
MAY BE USED INTERNALLY OR EXTERNALLY.

Mentals
Weariness.
Wants respect owed to them.

Modalities
Worse in warm, moist air.
Worse for pressure.
Worse for motion.
Better for rest.

Likes and dislikes
Likes cold drinks.

Disease tendencies
Varicose veins—knotty, swollen and sore.
Haemorrhoids which bleed freely.
Sensation of a weight in the rectum.
Chilblains.

Physical features
Bloodshot eyes, congested blood vessels on the cheeks and nose.

HEPAR SULPH

★★★★★

(Calcium sulphide)

SENSITIVE TO ALL IMPRESSIONS—touch, pain and cold.
PERSPIRES EASILY, both day and night, although always likes to keep well covered.
Any skin problem seems to SUPPURATE, or gather pus.
CATARRHAL TENDENCY.
There is CHILLINESS.
SPLINTER-LIKE PAINS, especially of the throat.

Mentals
Irritable at the slightest provocation.
'Touchy,' even to the point of ferociousness.
Easily offended.
Speaks quickly.

When angry can easily go over the top.
Grumbling nature.
Can be quite resentful.

Modalities
Worse for touch.
Worse for dry, cold winds.
Worse for draughts.
BETTER IN WET WEATHER.
BETTER FOR WRAPPING HEAD UP.
Better for eating.

Likes and dislikes
Likes pickles.
Likes vinegar.
Likes spices.
Dislikes fat.

Disease tendencies
Skin problems which lead to infections.
Bedsores.
Ulcers of the skin.
Sore throats with swollen glands.
Eye infections.

Physical features
Cracked lower lip.
Perspires freely, but keeps wrapped up in spite of this.
Perspiration may have sour, offensive odour.
Skin discharges also tend to be offensive.

HYPERICUM
(St John's Wort)

A great remedy for all puncturing or crushing injuries, e.g. treading on nails, needles, splinters, trapped fingers and toes.

SPASMS after injury.
NEURALGIAS.

Mentals
Melancholic.
Depression after wounds, injuries or operations.
Dislike of heights.

Modalities
Worse for cold.
Worse for damp.
Worse for fog.
Worse for movement.
Worse for touch.
Better for bending the head back.
BETTER FOR RUBBING.

Likes and dislikes
Thirsty.
Likes wine.

Disease tendencies
Wounds, punctures, crushes, concussions.
Coccydynia.
Haemorrhoids which are sensitive and bleed easily.
Neuralgia.

Physical features
Nil in particular.

IGNATIA
(St Ignatius Bean)

An excellent remedy for the ILL EFFECTS OF SHOCK, GRIEF OR FEAR.
Symptoms are often UNEXPECTED or CONTRADICTORY, e.g. sore throats better for swallowing

solids, indigestion better for eating, fevers better for keeping warm.
There is CHILLINESS.
There is great HYPERSENSITIVITY TO PAIN.
THROBBING, BURSTING and CRAMP-LIKE PAINS.

Mentals
Capricious—moods change rapidly and unexpectedly.
'Temperamentally mercurial.' Can flit from joy to depression and tearfulness extremely rapidly and almost without warning.
Anxiety.
Effects of GRIEF.
May sit and sigh a lot—even decades after the event.
Easily offended.

Modalities
Worse in the mornings.
Worse in cold and open air.
Worse after food.
Worse for coffee.
BETTER WHILE EATING.
Better for changing position.
Better for lying on affected part.
Better for heat and the sun.

Likes and dislikes
Dislikes brandy.
Dislikes coffee.
Dislikes tobacco.
Likes sour food.
Likes vinegar and acidic food.

Disease tendencies
Hysterical problems.
Continued difficulty swallowing, especially after a bereavement. This is the condition known as 'Globus

Hystericus,' when it is harder to swallow liquids than solids.
'Psychosomatic problems.'
Headaches, like a nail being driven into the skull.
Cramp-like pains.

Physical features
May have involuntary twitching around the mouth.

IPECACUANHA
(Ipecac root)

SPASMODIC PROBLEMS.
WET, SPASMODIC COUGHS.
CONSTANT NAUSEA, with retching or vomiting.

Mentals
Irritability.
Contemptuous of all sorts of things.
Always wants something 'different.'

Modalities
Worse for the damp.
Worse for lying down.
Better for the open air.
Better for closing the eyes.
Better for cold drinks.

Likes and dislikes
Dislikes food in general.

Disease tendencies
Respiratory problems.
Spasmodic and wet coughs.
Catarrhal problems which make one retch.
Bronchitis.

Headaches, as if the bones are being crushed.
Nose-bleeds

Physical features
Rings around the eyes.

*****

KALI PHOS
(Potassium phosphate)

THE NERVE SOOTHER.
Great PROSTRATION.
There is general WEAKNESS.
There is CHILLINESS.
There are yellow discharges.
PAIN IN LOWER NECK and BACK OF CHEST.

Mentals
Anxiety.
Dread.
General lethargy.
Dislikes having to meet people, although hates being alone.
Easily sinks into depression.
Very nervous, TIMID and shy.
Irritability when forced out of shell, or backed into a corner.
Nightmares.
Despondency.
Poor memory and concentration when upset.
Fear of NERVOUS BREAKDOWN.

Modalities
Worse for worry.
Worse for physical exertion.
Worse for excitement.
Worse for eating.

Better for heat.
Better for movement.

Likes and dislikes
Likes ice-cold drinks.
Likes sweets.
Likes sour food.

Disease tendencies
Tension headaches.
Dizziness from lying down.
Tinnitus.
Wet cough with yellow sputum.
Colds with yellow catarrh and nasal discharge.
Yellow diarrhoea coming on while eating.
Cystitis with yellow urine.

Physical features
Thin, pale and always seems to look ill.
Blushes when stressed.
Tendency to perspire over the face and head.
Complains of pain in lower neck.

*****

LACHESIS

(Bushmaster or Surukuku Snake Venom)

An excellent remedy for the menopause and after.
There is BLUENESS and PURPLISHNESS in all skin problems.
There is BLOATEDNESS—dislike of tight clothing or anything around the neck.
There is BURNING.
There is HYPERSENSITIVITY—to touch and noise.
TALKATIVE—tending to ramble on, constantly going off at tangents.
There is RESTLESSNESS.

Tendency towards LEFT-SIDED PROBLEMS, e.g. sore throats start on the left.

Mentals

May feel full of sins.
Never at the best in the morning.
Never felt right since the menopause.
Suspicious of people and of the spouse.
Jealousy.
Nightmares.
There is post-menopausal depression.
Temper tantrums—can be quite vitriolic and deliberately hurtful.
Ailments come after grief.

Modalities

WORSE FOR SLEEP—always sleep into an aggravation of symptoms.
Worse for touch.
Worse for pressure.
Worse for motion.
Worse for heat.
Worse for hot drinks.
WORSE IN THE SPRING.
WORSE IN CLOUDY, OVERCAST WEATHER.
Better for warm applications.
Better after discharges, e.g. of infection, or nose-bleeds.

Likes and dislikes

Likes coffee.
Likes alcohol.
Likes seafood.
Likes cold drinks.

Disease tendencies

Sore throats—blue or purplish appearance. They start on the left side. The pain is usually out of proportion to the symptoms.

Asthma.
Hot flushes.
Headaches are typically hammering, worse for pressure and for sleep. May even wake up with a headache.
Palpitations, constricting anginal pains and a sensation of bloatedness.
Varicose veins—very blue and bloated.
Haemorrhoids—when they are large, blue or purple.

Physical features

Blue or purplish face when ill.
Thin builds, maybe even seeming emaciated.
Pale face when well.

★★★★★

LYCOPODIUM

(Club Moss)

RIGHT-SIDED PROBLEMS.
Always looks older and more worried than years.
Symptoms worse between 4 p.m. and 8 p.m.
Hair may have gone grey or fallen out prematurely.
CUTTING AND BURNING PAINS.
There is CHILLINESS.

Mentals

Lack of self-confidence.
Anticipatory anxiety of events, yet when the time comes they usually cope very well.
Sensitive types.
Melancholia.
Fears of being alone, death, ghosts, crowds.
Dislikes meeting strangers.
Forgetful of words when writing.
Irritable on waking.
Irritated by little things.

Dislikes contradiction.

Modalities
Worse for heat.
Worse for hot applications.
Worse for over-eating.
Better for motion.
Better for being uncovered.
Better for small meals.

Likes and dislikes
Likes sweet food.
Likes warm drinks.
Dislikes meat.
Dislikes cheese.
Dislikes seafood.

Disease tendencies
Migraine.
Sore throats, starting on the right side, better for warm drinks.
Digestive problems, e.g. flatulence, stomach ulcers, gall stones.
Kidney stones.
Hardening of the arteries.
Psoriasis.
Restless legs.
Dry vagina.

Physical features
Worried frown on forehead.
Intellectual types, e.g. teachers, lawyers, doctors.
May have been prematurely grey or bald.
Thin face, neck, chest, but well-nourished abdomen.
Tendency to stoop.
Often complains of one foot being hot while the other is cold.

MAGNESIA PHOSPHORICA

(Magnesium phosphate)

RIGHT-SIDED PROBLEMS.
CRAMPING OR SPASMODIC PAINS.
There is exhaustion.
Dislike of mental exertion.

Mentals
Placid nature.
Tends to lament about the pains they have suffered.
Wooliness of thinking.

Modalities
Worse right side.
Worse for the cold.
Worse for touch.
Worse at night.
Better for warmth.
Better for pressure.
Better for rubbing.
Better for doubling-up.

Likes and dislikes
Likes cold drinks.

Disease tendencies
Neuralgias.
Right-sided facial pain.
Right-sided sciatica.
Abdominal cramps and colic.
Tremors of the hand.
General muscular weakness.
Spasmodic coughs.

Physical features
Tired looking, languid types.

***** MERCURIUS SOLUBILIS

(Black oxide of mercury)

There is WEAKNESS and WEARINESS of the limbs.
There is often a TREMOR and a tendency to STAMMER.
Infections are associated with glandular enlargement.
There is OFFENSIVENESS of all discharges.
There is ready PERSPIRATION which is offensive.
There is a metallic taste.
There is SENSITIVITY to TEMPERATURE CHANGES.
There are BURNING and CUTTING PAINS.

Mentals
General SLOWNESS of THOUGHT.
Poor memory.
Distrustful of others.
Fear of losing reason.

Modalities
Worse for perspiring.
Worse for warmth of bed.
Worse at night.
Worse for damp.
Worse for lying on right side.

Likes and dislikes
Likes cold drinks.

Disease tendencies
Sore throats with exudate and offensive breath.
Recurrent mouth problems.
Skin ulcers.
Bedsores.

Physical features
Offensive breath.
Flabby tongue showing the imprint of the teeth.
Poor mouth hygiene and spongy gums.
Skin moist from perspiration.
Face pale, dirty grey looking.

***** NATRUM MURIATICUM
(Salt)

There is CHILLINESS.
There may be a TREMOR.
Colds start with repeated sneezing.
There are SORE, CRAMPING and HAMMERING PAINS.

Mentals
Touchiness.
Depression.
Ill effects or ailments from GRIEF.
Wants to weep but the tears won't come.
Broods on past slights.
Resentment.
Irritated by little things.
Dislikes sympathy.
Moody with changing emotions.
Dreams of burglars.

Modalities
Worse in mornings.
Worse by the sea.
Worse for the sun.
Worse for thunderstorms.

Likes and dislikes
Craves salt.
Likes cold drinks.

Dislikes bread.

Disease tendencies
Cold sores.
Mouth ulcers.
Colds and respiratory infections.
Depression after grief or shock.
HAMMERING HEADACHES with preceding ZIG-ZAG VISION.
Palpitations.
Warts on hands and fingers.
Difficulty passing urine, especially if anyone is present.

Physical features
Mapped tongue.
Cracked lower lip.
Oily skin and fine oily hair.
Thin neck and thin build, despite good appetite.

***** NITRICUM ACIDUM
(Nitric acid)

General WEAKNESS, as with all 'acid' types.
There is CHILLINESS.
SPLINTER-LIKE PAINS.
Generalised SPIKINESS.

Mentals
Depression.
Despair.
INDIFFERENCE.
Suspiciousness.
Obstinacy.
Irritability.
Vindictiveness.
Sensitivity to noise, pain and touch.
Fear of death.

Modalities

Worse in the evenings and at night.
Worse for wind.
Worse for damp.
Worse for thunder.
Better for movement.

Likes and dislikes

Likes 'indigestible' food.
Likes salt.
Likes fat.

Disease tendencies

Tension headaches.
Mouth ulcers.
Sore throats which feel like splinters in the throat.
Respiratory infections with prickling sensation in the chest.
Offensive urine.
Constipation.
Anal fissures.
Haemorrhoids which have splinter-like pain persisting for long after the last motion was passed.
Warts which prickle, bleed and itch.

Physical features

Brown-eyed.
May have been dark-haired.
Dark-complexioned.
Cracks around the nose and mouth.

*****

NUX VOMICA

(Poison nut—contains strychnine)

Mainly a MALE REMEDY.
There is CHILLINESS.

There is HYPERSENSITIVITY—to noise, light and smell.
Ill effects of OVER-INDULGENCE—alcohol, rich food, coffee, tea, etc.
BURNING, CUTTING, ACHING and BURSTING PAINS.

Mentals
IRRITABILITY.
Quarrelsome.
Dislikes contradiction.
Melancholic.
Dislikes being touched.
Always in a hurry.
Critical of others, always finding fault.

Modalities
Worse in the mornings.
Worse in windy weather.
Worse 2 hours after food.
Worse in open air.
Worse for the sun.
Better in the evening.
Better for sleep.
Better in damp, wet weather.
Better for pressure.

Likes and dislikes
Likes fat.
Likes rich food.

Disease tendencies
Recurrent headaches and migraine.
Stomach problems—heartburn and indigestion.
Gastritis from over-indulgence.
Alcohol excess.
Hiccoughs.
Strangulated hernias.

Lumbago.
Constipation.

Physical features
Thin build.
Sedentary types who like 'good food, wine and company.'
Always in a hurry.

PETROLEUM
(Crude rock oil)

TRAVEL SICKNESS.
DRY, CRACKED SKIN PROBLEMS.
Symptoms come and go rapidly.

Mentals
Poor sense of direction.
Irritable.
Easily offended.
Sometimes feels as if he is a double of himself.
Fear of death.
Anxious to settle affairs.

Modalities
Worse for travel.
Worse for touch.
Worse for thunderstorms.
Better for warm air.
Better for lying well wrapped up.
Better for dry weather.

Likes and dislikes
Dislikes fat.

Disease tendencies
Dry, cracked skin.

Painful, itching chilblains.
Travel sickness.

Physical features
Dry skin with cracked fingertips.

PHOSPHORICUM ACIDUM
(Phosphoric acid)

There is general DEBILITY—mental first, followed by physical.
Ill effects of grief, disappointment and having 'overdone it.'

Mentals
Mild nature.
Apathy.
Indifference.
Poor memory and confusion after disappointment.

Modalities
Worse for exertion.
Worse for loss of body fluids, e.g. diarrhoea, perspiration, blood.
Worse for tight clothing.
Better for keeping warm.

Likes and dislikes
Likes juices.
Likes cold milk.
Dislikes sour things.

Disease tendencies
Inflamed eyes.
Effects of grief.
General debility and weakness.

Nose-bleeds.
Back pain between the shoulder blades.
Flatulence or very pale diarrhoea.

Physical features
May have gone grey or bald prematurely.
Blue rings around eyes.
Cracked lips.
Pale, earthy features.

*****

PHOSPHORUS
(Phosphorus)

HYPERSENSITIVITY of all the senses.
Tendency to bleed easily; bright red blood.
BURNING PAINS.
Symptoms come and go suddenly.
Low resistance to coughs, colds, gastric infections.
Perspires easily on exertion, or in the mornings (especially on the lower lip.)
There is CHILLINESS.
Emotions produce a TEMPERATURE.

Mentals
Artistic.
Intelligent.
Imaginative.
Psychic or clairvoyant.
Easily angered, flares up.
Fearful of things which creep and crawl, of thunderstorms, of the dark and death.
Restless and fidgety.
Depression.
Indifference.
Apathy.

Great fatigue.
Likes sympathy.
Likes to be sympathetic to others.
Constantly needs reassurance.

Modalities

Better for eating—may have to eat in the night.
Generally better for warmth, but head symptoms better for cold.
Better for rubbing.

Likes and dislikes

Likes salt.
Likes spices.
Likes sour food.
Likes cold drinks which may be vomited as they warm up in the stomach.
Worse lying on the left.

Disease tendencies

Glaucoma.
Styes.
Bleeding and bruising tendencies.
Vertigo.
Bursting headaches.
Recurrent respiratory infections.
Dry coughs.
Temperature and ailments after powerful emotions or excitement.

Physical features

Tall and slim.
Brown eyes with long eyelashes.
Pale skin and previously dark hair, or previously red-haired and freckled.
Tendency to perspire on upper lip.

***** # PULSATILLA

(The wind flower)

Usually a FEMALE REMEDY.
There is CHILLINESS.
CHANGEABLE and CONTRADICTORY SYMPTOMS, e.g. no two bouts of illness are the same; symptoms fluctuate hour by hour in a contradictory manner.
Perspiration on one side of the face.
NO THIRST.

Mentals
Mild and gentle.
Weeping tendency—for fear, misery or joy.
Laughs easily.
Tends to be quiet.
Likes sympathy.
Suspicious.
Jealous.
Irritable if slighted.
Religious nature. May feel full of sins.
Fear of the dark and of ghosts.

Modalities
Worse for a stuffy atmosphere.
Worse for heat.
Better up and about, although when ill may feel better lying well-propped up in bed.
Better for a good weep.
Better for the open air.
Better for sympathy or consolation.
Better for motion.

Likes and dislikes
Dislikes fat.
Dislikes rich food.

Disease tendencies
Styes.
Catarrhal problems.
Varicose veins.
Incontinence.
Irritable bowel.
Skin problems.

Physical tendencies
'Girlish appearance' despite age.
Fair-haired.
Blue-eyed.
Tendency to put on weight.

RANUNCULUS BULBOSUS
(Buttercup)

BRUISED or SORE PAINS.
Sensitive to air and touch.

Mentals
Nil in particular.

Modalities
Worse in open air.
Worse for motion.
Worse for touch.
Worse for changes in the weather.
Worse for stormy weather.

Likes and dislikes
Nil in particular.

Disease tendencies
Chest stitches.
Shingles.
Neuralgia following shingles (Post-herpetic neuralgia).

Blistering skin eruptions.
Itchy skin problems.
Chronic sciatica.

Physical features
Nil in particular.

RHODODENDRON
(Snow-rose)

An excellent rheumatic remedy.
ALWAYS WORSE BEFORE A STORM.
TEARING PAINS in neck and back.

Mentals
Dread of storms.
Fearful of thunder.
Poor memory generally.
Forgetful.

Modalities
Worse before storms.
All symptoms reappear in rough weather.
Better after storm breaks.
Better for warmth.
Better for eating.
Better immediately for moving.

Likes and dislikes
Nil in particular.

Disease tendencies
Headaches, eye-aches, toothaches, stitch-like chest pains, all of which are worse before a storm.
Arthritis worse before a storm.
Neuralgic pains of the face and teeth.

Physical features

Nil in particular.

RHUS TOXICODENDRON

(Poison ivy)

A great RHEUMATIC and SKIN remedy.

TEARING PAINS.

Mainly RIGHT-SIDED PROBLEMS.

Ill effects of getting wet or chilled while perspiring. Indeed, the ill effects of such an episode may have lingered for years.

There is RESTLESSNESS, so that the position has to be changed frequently.

Pains worse on starting to move, but get better as movement continues.

Stiffness on starting to move, but improving as movement continues.

Mentals

Melancholic.

Anxiety at night.

May contemplate suicide.

Modalities

Worse during sleep.

Worse during cold, wet weather.

Worse after rain.

Worse at night.

Worse lying on back.

Worse lying on right side.

Better for warmth.

Better for walking.

Better for changing position.

Better for rubbing.

Better for stretching.

Likes and dislikes
Likes milk.
Always thirsty.

Disease tendencies
Headaches after being in a draught or being chilled.
Inflamed eyes after being wet.
Joint pains better for movement.
Backache and lumbago.
Sprains and strains.
Sciatica.
Numbness and twitching of limbs.
Blistering skin problems.
Cold sores.
Shingles.

Physical features
Triangular red tip to the tongue.

RUTA GRAVEOLENS
(Rue)

A remedy for STRAINS.
PAINS as if BRUISED.

Mentals
Feels weak.
Despair.

Modalities
Worse lying down.
Worse for cold.
Worse for wetness.
Better for rubbing and scratching.

Likes and dislikes
Nil in particular.

Disease tendencies

Eye strain, from sewing, fine work or reading.
Headaches after over-doing it.
Backache and lumbago, better for lying on the back.
Painful wrists.

Physical features

Nil in particular.

★★★★★ SEPIA
(Cuttlefish ink)

Usually a FEMALE REMEDY.
DRAGGING DOWN SENSATION, as if the womb is about to prolapse. Often wants to cross the legs to get rid of the sensation.
May be very depressed and withdrawn, but COMES ALIVE WITH EXERTION, classically dancing.
There is CHILLINESS, although flushes are common.
BURNING OR THROBBING PAINS.

Mentals

SLOWNESS.
INDIFFERENCE to loved ones.
Depression.
Tiredness and weakness.
Aggression to loved ones.
Irritable and easily offended.
Weepiness.
Feels that cannot cope.
Wants to get away from it all.
Likes a good cry.
Dislikes sympathy and consolation.
Dislikes company, but hates being alone. Tends to avoid crowds.
Resentful of people who interfere or fuss after them.
Fear of disease.

Modalities
Worse for tobacco.
Worse before a storm.
Worse for too much sedentary work.
Better for food.
Better for exertion, especially dancing.
Better for sleep.

Likes and dislikes
Dislikes meat.
Dislikes milk.
Dislikes fat.
Likes vinegar.
Likes spices.

Disease tendencies
Depression, especially after the menopause.
Migraine and headaches, better for sleep.
Menopausal problems.
Constipation, with a ball-like sensation in the back passage.
Haemorrhoids.

Physical features
Thin build.
Yellowish 'saddle' across the bridge of the nose, or a 'butterfly' rosy colouration across the cheeks and nose.
Cracked lower lip.
May have been brunette.

***** SILICA
(Flint)

SLOW HEALING.
There is CHILLINESS.
There is offensive perspiration of the head and feet.
Prone to colds and respiratory infections.

BURNING, CUTTING, SORE AND THROBBING PAINS.

Mentals
Dread of failure.
Lack of self-confidence.
Timidity.
Anticipatory anxiety of events and appointments.
Exhausted after conversation.
Dislikes talking.
Fixed ideas about pins—wants to find them and count them.
Basically fears them.

Modalities
Worse for draughts.
Better for warmth.
Better for wrapping up.

Likes and dislikes
Likes cold food.
Always thirsty.
Dislikes meat.
Dislikes milk.

Disease tendencies
Boils and septic tendencies.
Bone pains and bone problems.
Headaches, better for wrapping up.
Chest infections that are slow to clear.
History of TB.
Constipation—when the motion can only be partially expelled and tends to slip back.

Physical features
Thin, delicate 'China-doll' appearance (prominent foreheads).
Small sweaty hands and feet.
White spots on the nails.

SPIGELIA
(Pinkroot)

A remedy of DEBILITY in anaemia and rheumatism.
There is CHILLINESS.
There is sensitivity to touch.

Mentals
Fear of sharp objects.

Modalities
Worse for touch.
Worse for motion.
Worse for noise.
Worse for washing.
Better for lying on the right side with the head propped high.
Better for breathing in.

Likes and dislikes
Nil in particular.

Disease tendencies
Glaucoma.
Facial neuralgias.
Palpitations and angina, and angina with palpitations.
Both of these heart symptoms seem to be relieved by drinking hot water.

Physical features
Pale, debilitated looking.

SPONGIA
(Roasted sponge)

FAMILY OR PERSONAL HISTORY OF TB.
Susceptibility to glandular involvement.

DRYNESS of symptoms—thus, dry cough, hoarse dry voice, dry passages.
CONSTRICTING SYMPTOMS.

Mentals
Anxiety and fears of all sorts. The worse are the fears, the worse do the other symptoms become, e.g. cough.

Modalities
Worse for climbing the stairs.
Worse for the wind.
Worse in the late evening.
Better for descending the stairs.
Better for eating and drinking.

Likes and dislikes
Always thirsty.

Disease tendencies
Dry cough.
Hoarse voice and recurrent respiratory infections.
Angina, worse after midnight.
Palpitations, such that there is the sensation that the heart could burst.
Hiccoughs.

Physical features
Nil in particular.

*****

STAPHISAGRIA
(Stavesacre)

AILMENTS FROM SUPPRESSED ANGER OR INDIGNATION.
HYPERSENSITIVE TO TOUCH.
Good remedy after any cuts, e.g. operations.

Mentals
Violent flare-ups of temper.
Aggressiveness.
Hypochondriacal—always thinking about their illness and their symptoms.
Very sensitive.
Easily offended.
Likes solitude.
Resentment.

Modalities
Worse for the cold.
Worse for touch.

Likes and dislikes
Likes tobacco.
Likes milk.

Disease tendencies
Depression.
Good post-operative remedy to hasten healing after the body has been cut or incised.
Headaches from anger or strong emotions.
Styes.
Colic after anger.
Prostate enlargement.
Eczema.
Warts around the back passage.
Skin problems which start after anger.

Physical features
Sunken eyes, itchy, flaky eyelids. May have eczema with thickish crusts.

*****

SULPHUR
(Sulphur)

BURNING OR ITCHING.
REDNESS of affected parts.

OFFENSIVENESS OF ODOURS.

DIRTINESS—there will always be at least one aspect of the appearance which has been left. For example, if a nice new suit is worn, the shoes may be left unpolished. Neatness and cleanliness is not high on their order of priorities.

There is PERIODICITY, in that symptoms seem to come on every seven days during an illness.

Skin complaints alternate with internal problems.

There is FIDGETING—they are unable to stand, sit or lie still. They have to lean, change feet, etc.

There is general HOTNESS.

Mentals

Philosophical nature.

Selfish and self-centred.

Argumentative and aggressive.

Sensitive to odours, although they themselves may have offensive perspiration which they are oblivious to.

Dislike getting washed or bathed, although may be fond of swimming.

Modalities

Worse for washing or bathing.

Worse for the heat of the bed.

Worse at 11 a.m., when gets a sinking feeling in the stomach.

Worse for standing or sitting still.

Better for the open air.

Likes and dislikes

Always thirsty.

Always hungry.

Likes fat.

Likes sweets.

Likes coffee and other stimulants.

Likes alcohol.

Disease tendencies

Glaucoma.
Catarrhal problems.
Skin problems of all sorts.
BURNING PAINS.
Burning feet.
Early morning diarrhoea which makes them get out of bed.
Constipation.
Haemorrhoids—red, burning and itching.
Lumbago on getting up in the morning or when turning.
Alcoholism.
Gout.

Physical features

Red-lipped.
Dirty appearance.
Lean, lanky, 'ragged philosopher' appearance.
Sometimes may be more like a well-rounded bon viveur.
Always leaves at least one article of clothing, or one aspect of appearance unkempt.

THUJA OCCIDENTALIS
(Arbor vitae)

A great WART REMEDY.
There is CHILLINESS.
There is a sweet odour to the perspiration which is often profuse over uncovered parts.

Mentals

Anxiety.
Weeps easily.
Makes mistakes in reading and writing.
Can get odd ideas fixed in their minds, e.g. as if the body is rigid, brittle like glass. As if something is living inside them.

Modalities
Worse for the heat of the bed.
Worse at night.
Worse for cold.

Likes and dislikes
Dislikes potatoes.
Dislikes meat.
Dislikes fat.
LOVES TEA.

Disease tendencies
Headaches, as if a nail is being driven into skull.
Styes.
Nasal polyps.
Haemorrhoids.
Nail problems.
Warts and warty growths anywhere.

URTICA URENS

(Stinging-nettle)

BURNING and STINGING PAINS.
BLISTERING ERUPTIONS.

Mentals
Nil in particular.

Modalities
Worse for water.
Worse for touch.
Worse for scratching.
Better for rubbing.
Better for lying down.

Likes and dislikes
Nil in particular.

Disease tendencies
Urticaria, a blistering or raised weal skin condition with intense itching, just like a nettle-rash.
Arthritic pains which alternate with episodes of urticaria.

ZINCUM METALLICUM
(Zinc)

SENSITIVE TO NOISES AND TALKING.
RESTLESS LEGS.
There is CHILLINESS.
CRAMPING PAINS.
Lack of vitality.
Twitching tendency.
Anaemia is common.

Mentals
Depression.
Poor memory.
Feels as if the head will fall to one side, because it is so heavy.

Modalities
Worse after dinner.
Worse for wine.
Better while eating.
Better after discharges, from nose, wounds etc.

Likes and dislikes
Always hungry in late morning, with a ravenous appetite.

Disease tendencies
Chilblains.
Cramps of all sorts.
Varicose veins.
Restless legs.

Therapeutic Index

An A–Z of common symptoms and conditions and the remedies most likely to help.

ACIDITY—Calc carb, Mag phos, Nux vom.

AGGRESSIVENESS—Bell, Nux vom, Staph, Sulph.

ALCOHOL, ILL EFFECTS—Ars alb, Bar carb, Nux vom, Sulph.

ALUMINIUM, ILL EFFECTS—Alum. (See Chapter 8)

ANAEMIA—there are several different types of anaemia, all of which necessitate a specific diagnosis. Once this has been made, the following might be of use.

—Ars alb, Ferr, Chin, Nat mur.

ANGER—Acon, Coloc, Hep sulph, Ign, Nux vom, Staph. (See Chapter 6)

ANGINA—Cact, Lach, Spig, Spon. (See Chapter 11)

ANUS, ITCHING—Alum, Amb gris, Nit ac, Sulph.

ANXIETY—See under APPREHENSION and FEARS. (See Chapter 6)

APATHY—Apis, Chin, Nat mur, Phos, Puls, Sep. (See Chapter 6)

APPETITE, POOR—a sustained loss of appetite can be a significant symptom which needs investigation. A temporary loss of appetite might respond to the following.

—Calc carb, Nux vom, Lyc, Puls, Rhus tox.

APPREHENSION—Arg nit, Ars alb, Gels, Lyc, Sil. (See Chapter 6)

ARTHRITIS—Apis, Arg nit, Arn, Bry, Caust, Dulc, Puls, Rhod, Rhus, Rut, Sulph. (See Chapters 9 & 10)

BACKACHE—Acon, Arn, Bry, Calc carb, Dulc, Nux vom, Phos ac, Rhod, Rhus. (See Chapters 9 & 10)

BEDSORES—Ars alb, Bell, Lach, Nit ac, Sil. (See Chapter 15)

BEREAVEMENT (See Chapter 6)

BLISTERING SKIN ERUPTIONS—If large or painful a medical opinion should be sought.

—Ars alb, Caust, Lach, Nat mur, Nit ac, Phos, Ranunc, Rhus tox.

BOILS—Apis, Arn, Ars alb, Graph, Hep sulph, Lach, Sil.

BORING PAINS—Arg nit, Bell, Puls, Spig. (See Chapter 9)

BREASTS, HEAVY OR ACHING—a medical opinion should always be sought.

—Bry, Lach. (See Chapter 14)

BRONCHITIS—Acon, Ars alb, Bry, Ipec, Puls, Sulph.

BRUISES—Arn, Hamam, Hyper, Rut. (See Chapter 16)

BURNING PAINS—Acon, Apis, Arn, Ars alb, Bell,

Bry, Caust, Euph, Graph, Merc, Nat mur, Nit ac, Nux vom, Phos, Phos ac, Puls, Rhus tox, Spig, Sulph. (See Chapter 9)

BURNS—Caust, Hamam.

CATARRH—Aur, Graph, Hep sulph, Nat mur, Sulph.

CHANGING SYMPTOMS—Puls.

CHILBLAINS—Apis, Ars alb, Calc carb, Graph, Hamam, Petrol, Puls, Rhus tox, Zinc.

COCCYDYNIA (PAIN IN COCCYX)—Apis, Caust, Hyper.

COLD (COMMON)—Acon, Euph, Gels, Nat mur, Puls.

COLD SORES—Dulc, Nat mur, Ranun, Rhus tox.

COLIC—Coloc, Cup met, Mag phos, Staph.

CONFUSION—Alum, Amb gris, Anac, Apis, Bar carb, Caust, Cocc, Lyc, Rhod. (See Chapter 8)

CONJUNCTIVITIS—Acon, Aur, Arg nit, Ars alb, Bell, Dulc, Euph, Rhus tox.

CONSOLATION, WORSE FOR—Ign, Nat mur, Sep.
BETTER FOR—Puls.

CONSTIPATION—Any alteration in bowel habit which is sustained needs a medical opinion. (See Chapter 12)

—Alum, Bry, Bar carb, Calc carb, Nit act, Sep, Sulph, Sil.

CONSTRICTING PAINS—Cact, Coloc, Cup met, Phos.

CONTRACTURES OF TENDONS AND MUSCLES —Caust.

CORNS—Arn, Calc carb, Lyc, Sil, Sulph.

COUGH (See Chapter 11)

DRY, NON-PRODUCTIVE—Acon, Bar carb, Bell, Bry, Calc carb, Puls, Phos, Spon.

WET, PRODUCTIVE—Dulc, Ipecac, Merc, Sep.

SPASMODIC—Cocc, Cup met, Ipecac, Mag phos.

CRACKED LIPS—Graph, Hep sulph, Nat mur, Phos ac, Sep.

CRAMP PAINS—Bell, Caust, Calc carb, Coloc, Cup met, Mag phos, Nat mur, Phos, Phos ac, Sulph, Zinc. (See Chapter 9)

CYSTITIS—If sustained, then a medical opinion should be sought.

—Apis, Arg nit, Ars alb, Bar carb, Bell, Caust, Dulc, Kali phos, Nux vom, Puls, Sep, Sulph.

DEAFNESS—Caust, Chin, Nit ac, Puls, Sil. (See Chapter 8)

DEBILITY—If sustained a medical opinion should be sought. If merely found to be run down, then the following may help.

—Arn, Ars alb, Calc carb, Kali phos, Nux vom, Sep.

DEPRESSION—Anac, Ars alb, Aur, Calc carb, Ign, Lyc, Nat mur, Puls, Staph, Sulph. (See Chapter 6)

DESPAIR—Acon, Ars alb, Bry, Calc carb, Nux vom, Sep. (See Chapter 6)

DIARRHOEA—Any alteration in bowel habit which is sustained needs a medical opinion. (See Chapter 12)

—Arg nit, Ars alb, Bry, Coloc, Gels, Lyc, Puls, Sulph.

DIZZINESS (and VERTIGO)—Bell, Bry, Calc carb, Chin, Cocc, Ferr met, Gels, Kali phos, Nat mur, Puls.

DREAMS, FEARFUL—Acon, Alum, Ars alb, Bar carb, Calc carb, Nat mur, Phos, Puls, Thuj.

OF BEING CHASED—Sil, Sulph.

OF THE DEAD—Ars alb, Thuj.

DREAMS OF FLYING—Apis.

OF MURDER—Arn, Nat mur, Petrol.

DRY SKIN—Alum, Calc carb, Graph, Nit ac, Nat mur, Petrol, Sulph. (See Chapter 15)

DYSPHAGIA (DIFFICULTY SWALLOWING)—Chin, Gels, Ign, Lach, Nit ac. (See Chapter 12)

EARACHE—Apis, Bell, Lach, Nit ac, Nux vom, Puls, Sulph.

EXCITEMENT, ILLNESS AFTER—Acon, Arg nit, Aur, Coff, Graph, Nat mur, Phos ac.

EYESTRAIN—Rut.

FEARS (See Chapter 6)

OF CROWDS—Acon, Arg nit, Lyc.

OF DARK—Acon, Calc carb, Caust, Cup met, Lyc, Puls.

OF DEATH—Acon, Apis, Arg nit, Ars alb, Bell, Bry, Calc carb, Caust, Coff, Cup met, Gels, Hep sulph, Lach, Lyc, Nux vom, Phos ac, Phos, Puls, Rhus tox.

OF GHOSTS—Acon, Ars alb, Caust, Lyc, Phos, Puls, Sulph.

OF HEIGHTS—Arg nit, Hyper.

OF INCURABLE ILLNESS—Phos, Sep.

OF NOISE—Caust.

OF PEOPLE—Acon, Ars alb, Aur, Bar carb, Lyc, Nat mur, Puls, Rhus tox.

OF STORMS—Nat mur, Rhod.

FEET, BURNING—Graph, Phos, Puls, Sulph.

GLAUCOMA—This is a condition which must be treated medically. The following may help.

—Gels. Rut

GOUT—Lyc, Puls.

GRIEF—Aur, Caust, Ign, Nat mur, Phos ac, Puls. (See Chapter 6)

HAEMORRHOIDS—Aloe, Bar carb, Caust, Hamam, Hyper, Nit ac. (See Chapter 12)

HANDS, CRACKED—Alum, Calc carb, Nat mur, Petrol, Sep, Sil, Sulph.

HEADACHE—Sudden severe headache must be treated seriously in view of the danger of strokes. Similarly, if sustained a medical opinion should be sought.

BURSTING—Bell, Bry, Chin, Lach, Nat mur, Phos, Sep.

LIKE A NAIL BEING DRIVEN IN—Coff, Ign, Thuj.

THROBBING—A sustained throbbing headache must be considered to be caused by temporal arteritis until proven otherwise. A medical opinion should be sought urgently since this condition can lead to blindness if untreated. (See Chapter 10)

—Bell, Chin, Nat mur, Lyc, Sulph.

TIGHT—Apis, Caust, Gels.

HEART PROBLEMS—See ANGINA. (See Chapter 11)

HEARTBURN—Calc carb, Lyc, Nux vom, Puls. (See Chapter 12)

HICCOUGH—Ars alb, Ign, Ipecac, Mag phos, Nux vom, Ranun, Spon.

HOARSE VOICE—If sustained beyond two weeks then a medical opinion should be sought to exclude dangerous conditions affecting the larynx.

—Caust, Dros, Phos.

HYSTERIA—Aur, Caust, Gels, Ign, Lach, Nat mur, Puls, Sep.

INCONTINENCE—Apis, Caust, Nat mur, Sep. (See Chapter 13)

INDIFFERENCE—Apis, Chin, Nat mur, Phos, Puls, Sep. (See Chapter 6)

INDIGESTION—Arg nit, Nux vom, Puls, Sulph. (See Chapter 12)

INJURIES—Acon, Arn, Hyper. (See Chapter 16)

INSOMNIA—Arn, Ars alb, Bell, Chin, Coff, Ign, Nux vom, Phos, Spig, Sulph. (See Chapter 7)

INSUFFICIENT INTEREST IN PRESENT CIRCUMSTANCES—(See Chapter 6)

INTOLERANCE OF PAIN—Coff, Phos.

ITCHING—Alum, Anac, Ars alb, Calc carb, Graph, Sulph, Urt. (See Chapter 15)

JEALOUSY—Apis, Lach, Puls. (See Chapter 6)

JOINT PAINS—Apis, Bry, Rhod, Rhus tox, Rut.

LACK OF CONFIDENCE (See Chapter 6)

LARYNGITIS—See HOARSENESS. If sustained beyond two weeks then a medical opinion should be sought to exclude dangerous conditions affecting the larynx.

—Acon, Arg nit, Bell, Dros, Gels, Hep sulph, Phos, Rhus tox, Spon.

LONELINESS (See Chapter 6)

LOVE, EFFECTS OF DISAPPOINTED (EVEN FIFTY YEARS LATER)—Aur, Ign, Lach, Nat mur.

LUMBAGO—See BACKACHE.

MEMORY PROBLEMS—Alum, Amb gris, Anac, Apis, Bar carb, Cocc, Lyc, Rhod. (See Chapter 8)

METALLIC TASTE—Cup met, Merc.

MOUTH ULCERS—Hep sulph, Nat mur, Nit ac.

NAIL PROBLEMS—Petrol.

NASAL POLYPS—Calc carb, Puls, Thuj

NAUSEA—Ars alb, Calc carb, Cocc, Cup met, Ipecac, Nux vom, Puls.

NEURALGIA—Acon, Ars alb, Coloc, Hyper, Mag phos, Ranun, Spig.

NOISE, SENSITIVE TO—Acon, Bell, Chin, Coff, Nux vom, Sep.

NOSE BLEEDS IF RECURRENT—Hamam, Ipecac, Phos.

OFFENDED EASILY—Alum, Apis, Ars alb, Aur, Calc carb, Caust, Chin, Graph, Lyc, Nux vom, Petrol, Puls, Sep, Spig.

OVER-CONCERN FOR WELFARE OF OTHERS (See Chapter 6)

OVER-SENSITIVE TO INFLUENCES AND IDEAS (See Chapter 6)

OVER-SENSITIVE TO SMELLS—Acon, Aur, Chin, Coff, Ign, Lyc, Nux vom, Phos, Sep.

PAIN (See Chapter 9)

PALPITATIONS—Ars alb, Bar carb, Nat mur, Rhus tox, Spig. (See Chapter 11)

PANIC (See Chapter 6)

PARALYTIC PROBLEMS—All such conditions must be diagnosed by a professional. Once diagnosed the following may be of help.

—Ars alb, Bar carb, Cup met.

PROSTATE PROBLEMS—A medical opinion is essential if there is any suspicion of a prostate problem in men. Once diagnosed as benign the following may be of help.

—Bar carb, Calc carb, Sil. Thuj (See Chapter 13)

RASHES (See Chapter 15)

RHEUMATISM (See Chapter 10)

SCIATICA—Ars alb, Coloc, Lyc, Mag phos, Rhus tox (See Chapter 10)

SHINGLES—Ars alb, Lach, Ranun, Thuj. (See Chapter 15)

SINUSITIS—Bell, Calc carb, Hep sulph, Puls, Spig.

SKIN PROBLEMS (See Chapter 15)

SLEEP PROBLEMS—See INSOMNIA. (See Chapter 7)

SMELL, DIMINISHED SENSE OF—Anac, Calc carb, Nat mur, Phos, Puls. (See Chapter 8)

SORE THROAT—Arg nit, Bell, Gel, Hep sulph, Nit ac, Nux vom, Puls.

SPRAINS—Acon, Arn, Calend. (See Chapter 16)

STOMACHACHE—Chin, Graph, Hep sulph, Ign, Phos, Sep, Sulph.

STYES—Graph, Phos, Puls, Staph, Thuj.

TASTE, METALLIC—Cup met, Merc.

TINNITUS—Caust, Chin. (See Chapter 8)

TONGUE—Pale tongues may indicate anaemia, so a medical opinion should be sought

PATTERNED—Nat mur.

TRIANGULAR RED TIP—Rhus tox.

TRAVEL SICKNESS—Acon, Cocc, Petrol.

TREMORS—Since this may herald the onset of cerebrovascular disease or Parkinson's disease, a medical opinion should be sought.

—Gels, Ign, Mag phos, Merc, Nat mur.

ULCERATION OF THE SKIN—Ars alb, Bell, Lach, Nit ac, Sil. (See Chapter 15)

UNCERTAINTY (See Chapter 6)

URINE PROBLEMS (See Chapters 13 & 14)

URTICARIA (NETTLE RASH)—Urt.

VAGINAL DRYNESS—Hamam, Lyc, Nat mur, Nit ac, Sulph. (See Chapter 14)

VARICOSE VEINS—Arn, Hamam, Puls.

VERTIGO—See DIZZINESS.

VOMITING—Ars alb, Cup met, Ipecac, Nux vom.

WARTS—Calc carb, Caust, Nat mur, Nit ac, Thuj. (See Chapter 15)

WEEPINESS—Apis, Ign, Nat mur, Puls, Sep. (See Chapter 6)

WOUNDS (See Chapter 16)

Index

Using the Index

Physical symptoms, feelings and emotions all play their part in homoeopathic diagnosis. The entries in this index use the words shown in the text and have been cross referenced to similar and related terms, but if the particular word you are looking for is not listed please look up a similar term (e.g. crying is not listed but tearfulness and weepiness are). Sub-headings have been used to break up long lists of page numbers so the relevant entry can be found quickly but sometimes this has been impossible (e.g. chilliness). In this case I would suggest looking up another symptom first. All major entries are shown in bold.